More Middle Age Madness

My menopause diary

By

Sarah Stenton

Dedication

This book is for my girls, Holly and Ella, lovely, kind, strong young women who put up with their mother writing about her menopause all over social media.

To those ladies who feel alone and unheard: This book is for you, I hope it gives you the voice you have been searching for.

And to my grandmother and the generations before me: Thank you for giving us the courage to speak out and stand up for better understanding and proper treatment of the menopause.

Acknowledgements

Thank you to all the people who follow my Facebook page for your unwavering support. I am so proud of the lovely, slightly crazy family we have created.

With love to my friends, my mum, dad and sister, and my much better half, David.

And finally, thanks to the menopause for being such a ball ache it has given me enough material to write this book!

About the author

Sarah was born in Oxford in 1971, has lived in Manchester and France and now lives in Shropshire with her husband, two daughters and two dogs.
She has published one previous book; 'Middle age madness, my menopause diary' which is available on Amazon and Kindle, and this book is the second installment of the series.

You can follow Sarah's page, 'middle age madness' on Facebook for day-to-day updates on life in the middle age lane.

Introduction

Whilst gathering material for this book I found some previously unpublished diary entries that take us to just before the pandemic and out of the other side.
Although this book is primarily about 2023, I have included these older entries because they reminded me just how tough lockdown was on all of us, and the different ways I found to try and cope.
That said, this is, overall, a lighthearted look at the menopause and some of the more surprising side effects that I have experienced.
Join me as I face the challenges that only the menopause can bring: who knew stair gates and sneezes could create such terror?
Will I ever find my sex drive again?
And what is a Moregasm?
Read on to find out more…

Spare me

15th June 2019

Friday evening, I made a red Thai chicken curry, it smelt delicious and I was starving.

Husband popped upstairs to change out of workwear. Being a porker, I decided not to wait for him and started to inhale my curry. I had underestimated by some degree how hot the fucker was and instantly started choking.

My body obviously decided I was dying and, to make sure I choked to death with maximum class and dignity, I pissed myself on the sofa.

Thankfully, I did not pass away, and, when I surfaced spluttering back into my body, I realised I had two choices: Let my dinner go cold and clean myself up or pretend the great piss flood had never happened and carry on eating.

To spare my dignity and avoid having to admit that I had piddled everywhere, I, in an admittedly poor token show of self-pride, sprayed myself liberally with Febreze and then sprayed the room slightly more enthusiastically.

Husband came down and sniffed appreciatively, it smells nice in here he said.

Febreze flavoured curry with under hints of piss must be a thing in his world.

I bolted my curry down and disappeared to the kitchen, stripped off from the waist down and shoved everything I had peed on in the washing machine.

This was much to the surprise of a passing horse rider who, glancing into my kitchen, got an eyeful of bum and a winking arse hole hastily shoving jeans into the washing machine.

So much for sparing my dignity.

22nd June 2019
Church or Chapel

Yesterday was a lovely day, my friend Mrs A and I had a spa day.
Mrs A is a lovely olive-skinned colour. I have an attractive skin tone somewhere between clay, chalk and putty.
Naturally I had spent the night before slathering Dove summer glow all over my newly shaved body.
I say body because, let's be honest, I basically have to shave the entire length of me these days.
Like I am a primate.
Just to be sure that I would look as glowing and lovely as Mrs A, I applied a final slathering of Dove on the morning of our spa day.
I looked at the clock and realised I was running late.
Therefore, the summer glow was not quite dry when I shoved my jeans on.
The was evident when I got undressed and had had 'Next Denimwear size 16' imprinted on my arse, along with the stencilled marks of seams and pockets.
Sometimes you just cannot win, and I feel I need to learn this lesson sooner rather than later.
We sat around the pool having a natter then did some serious exercising by leaning over to pick up a magazine.
'HOW HOT IS YOUR VAGINA?' screamed Cosmo, much to our middle age surprise.
We both agreed our vaginas were very hot, especially at night when one is sweating ones flaps off. But I don't think that is what Cosmo had in mind.
No doubt there were referring to having a bejazzled fanny or some sort of procedure where you can tighten up your hoof.

If you stuck some sort of embellishment on my vag to bejazzle the old girl, it would be lost in the undergrowth by Thursday.

We had lunch and a bottle of fizz then went in for our treatments.

As soon as I lay down, I needed to fart, courtesy of the fizz bubbles.

An interesting battle of wills commenced: my masseuse was trying to prise my bum cheeks apart – I don't know why; I had not paid for extras – and I was trying to keep my cheeks firmly closed to stop myself blowing the doors off the spa. My stomach inflated with unfarted gas, and I rose higher and higher on the bed.

At one pint my lady was on tip toes straining to reach me. Finally, mercifully, she left the room and I released, obliterating the delightful scent of oils and lotions from the room. When she came back in, she sniffed with distaste and went to check the drains.

Better out than in. As my grandad used to say: wherever you be let your wind go free, whether in church or chapel, let your rectum rattle.

I didn't really stand much chance of being ladylike, did I?

The changing room
Sunday August 18th 2019
I went into town yesterday and saw there was a sale on in a
shop I have thus far considered too middle aged. To my
equal surprise and horror, I found myself walking in and
touching things.
I even touched a crochet top!
I toyed with a neck scarf but quickly put it back.
A twinset caught my eye so I marched on, pretending I had
not seen it.
I stopped and touched a cardigan I thought would look nice
to wear round the garden centre and shook my head to try
and shake off the image.
I tried to like semi-trendy things like combat pants but was
drawn to the jeggings section. Practical and comfortable.
I avoided anything with a zip and wondered how long ago it
was that I willingly purchased a dress or something that
zipped up?
Trying to inch a zip slowly up and over back fat whilst
holding your breath and melting your flaps off is not much
fun.
Even if you manage to get the damn thing zipped up your
stomach sticks out so far you look full term pregnant, so you
immediately have to take the dress off again. You then have
the reverse torture of trying to lift your ham arms over your
head to grasp the top of the zip and try to drag it down.
More often than not you are so flushed and sweaty that the
item clings to you like a second skin and refuses to budge.
The law of middle age dictates that if you do manage to find
something you like enough to take into the changing rooms,
the lighting and mirrors will make you look the absolute
worst version of yourself.
And you will have massive dishcloth grey pants on complete
with piss pad and a bra that is best described as comfortable.

In reality, it has no support, is 15 years old, doubles as a
duster, gives you a shelf of back fat, and your boobs splay
out in opposite directions to their default position of under
each arm pit.

Despite your optimism, the items you take in will be too
fucking small and your arse crack will try and chew the
changing room curtain.

Instead of feeling beautiful and pleased with yourself you
spend the whole time trying to avoid looking at yourself in
the mirror, yanking cubicle curtain out of your hole and
praying your farts come out as silent ones.

Whenever I pluck up the courage to brave the changing
room, there is always some cow in there with her poor fat
friend, saying something like 'Oh, can you get me a size 6
please, Donna? This size 8 absolutely drowns me'

Or: 'Oh No, I look enormous in this size 10, I'm soooo fat!'
All said as I am trying to squeeze my legs into size 16 jeans
using Vaseline and a shoe horn. I feel like waddling out there
with the jeans straining round my thighs saying 'kiss my big
old arse, bitch, and shut up' but instead, I exit the changing
room with a dozen other ladies, looking flustered and
defeated and shoot a murderous glance towards cubicle
number 4.

Then I buy a pair of lovely, comfortable jeggings and walk
quickly out of the shop before my fart catches up with me.

The List

October 30th 2019

I have decided to make a list of things that annoy me:

Pubic Hair - Why has it been outlawed? Almost as soon as it starts to grow it is removed with all haste never to been seen again until you are too fat to find it or too lazy to care.

Eyebrows - Why do young girls have them four shades darker and as thick as caterpillars?

Chin Hair - Why? I did not ask for it, I do not want it and I cannot get rid of the fecking stuff.

Pelvic Floor - Where did it go the minute I turned 45 years old?

The Constant Fart - Why do I need to fart myself up out of a chair and puff my way across the room?

Countryfile - Why am I excited when it comes on?

Eyesight - Why does it start to fade just as I need it the most? How can I manage beard/moustache/cheek/nose hair pruning if I am losing the ability to see? Am I meant to have a hairy face?

Patience - Where has is gone? Why am I a snarling ball of fury?

Mammograms - You can bet your flaps that if men had to have their bollocks stretched, flattened, squeezed, and squashed between two metal plates someone would come up with a better way to carry out this test.

(Lovely staff though and very necessary)

Sex Drive - Why am I 'Noooo Matron' one minute and a raving nympho the next?

Garden centres and seed catalogues – Why? What is happening to me? Do they have some kind of magnetic pull that is impossible to resist once you reach middle age?

Clothes sizes – Why is a size 14 OK in one shop but in another you cannot get a pair of jeans in the same size over

your knee? Why am I a size 20 in one shop and a size 12 in another? It is a head wreck.
Memory - Why can't I remember what else I wanted to put on this list?

Thirsty Work.

Thursday 19th March 2020

Last night I decided to have a bath and then weigh myself. Bear in mind I have been doing OK with the diet and have a check in every week. I was expecting a nice little 2lb loss. My bath was lovely, I put loads of extra bubbles in to hide the rolls of flab in case husband should pop his head round the door and wonder why his wife had turned into a sumo wrestler

I had a coffee, read my book, and wallowed for an hour or so. I even shaved myself from the eyeballs down.

Out I got, dried off, spent approximately another hour chasing my shaven hair round the fucking bath and forcing it down the plug hole for husband to deal with later (blue job) and then I stood on the scales.

Horror of horror I had put on weight for the first time since starting this diet. I lashed around for something to blame other than the fact that I might be a greedy fucker, and, inexplicably, I made the decision that I had obviously fanny swallowed gallons of bathwater causing fluid retention and thus my weight had increased.

Yes, I would literally rather assume that my fandango hoovers up bathwater than admit that the ice cream I ate out of sheer boredom was the culprit.

Welcome to my world.

Happy Clappy

Saturday March 21st 2020

Yesterday husband and I hired a van to drive down to Bath and move our daughter out of university, it is closing in light of Covid-19.

Last time I saw my daughter's room at the halls of residence, we had just unpacked her to settle her in and it was clean and lovely.

In anticipation of a long day, husband and I packed a picnic to have with daughter when we arrived.

Holy Mary.

The smell sent us reeling.

By all accounts my offspring had been sick some three weeks previously and had been unable to locate the vomit in her festering bedroom.

'Get that fucking food away from here!' I hissed at husband, who was standing on the landing with our lovely wicker hamper.

Student halls of residence are no place for Waitrose picnic nibbles.

I will spare you the horror, but we got her packed up and the room cleaned and, suffice to say, we must both now be immune to every God-awful germ or bug known to man or beast.

*

The average age of male customers in my office is 79 so the other day when a real live action man helicopter pilot came in, I got very excited.

Husband took this heart, conveniently forgetting that every time an attractive lady come in, she goes out wearing his eyeballs glued to her back. (At such moments I am just 'Sarah.' For action man I suddenly became 'my wife Sarah' I thought he might actually piss on me at one point to lay his scent).

Anyway, husband wore a tight navy T shirt down to Bath,
with his new bum hugging jeans, occasionally muttering
'could've been a pilot but I chose Estate Agency' under his
breath as he drove.
I eyed husband up in the van, I eyed him up during the great
clean, I eyed him up removing furniture and I eyed him up
on the drive back to Shropshire.
I eyed him up in the bedroom. I was starkers.
Finally, he cottoned on.
He said he thought I looked nice too and you could see I had
lost weight. Foreplay done; he turned his back to whip his
jeans off.
I did a little shimmy of happiness.
As I shimmied, husband, who had his back still turned said
'are you giving yourself a round of applause?'
Alas, my hands were 3 ft apart mid shimmy.
My flaps were still clapping though.
Ah well.

Worry

March 25th 2020

I am writing this to you from my bedroom which has now been turned into an office because we had to close down our High Street office after the lock down announcement on Monday evening 23rd March.

It was a bit of a rush to get everything we needed packed up and, alas, we both forgot about bringing a chair.

The only spare chair at home is an ex-office one with a spitefully defunct gas compressor which will occasionally and alarmingly force the chair to crash to the floor.

Which is where I sit now with my arms extended above my head bashing about on the keyboard and hoping at least one word in three makes sense.

Just in case you had not quite got the message that this is pretty much rock bottom for your business, your fucking chair slams your arse down on the floor as if to prove the point.

Still, we are all healthy and well and that is what matters. But it is a very worrying time for all of us.

Luckily, husband and I work together so we are used to being together all the time and know exactly when to avoid each other like the pox.

For example, husband, worried about his business and the income being cut off overnight, has taken to sawing and chopping down every living thing in our garden, except the chickens.

Perhaps he will build us a little wooden cabin like Pa in Little House on the Prairie. I can be Ma and wear a bonnet with a lovely ribbon to hide my chin hair, and my two teenage daughters can have pretty plaits and kill each other in a loft bedroom.

It is a worrying and anxious time.

I am sure an awful lot of you are feeling the same.

One small positive note to end on, last night I had a lovely dream where husband had to go and find work as a stripper, and I rode in a lift - in every sense of the word - with James Martin. I could not quite meet his eye when watching him whisk his batter on TV this morning. I hope he washed his hands. He is a naughty boy!
Next time James, take the bracelet off, I worry it will get tangled up in my growler, and I've got quite enough to worry about as it is!

Pimm's and pain

Friday 3rd July 2020

Why do I have a pain in my right hip the very minute I crawl into bed? Am I so large that I am crushing my hip bone? Why is it just one side and not the other? Luckily, I prefer to lie on my left but alas, this puts me facing my husband and his fucking magnified breathing.

The inconsiderate bastard falls asleep the minute his head touches the pillow, knob and bollocks dangling dangerously and temptingly close to my knee. We have tried swapping sides of the bed but it just doesn't feel right. I have to have my side and he has to have his side. And so, I lie on my good hip waiting for sleep to come. I close my eyes and drift away at approximately 3.04 in the morning.

At approximately 3.06 I am nudged awake by a grumpy husband, himself roused out of a fine 5 hours sleep, because I have had the nerve to let out a lonely little snore. Being a loving and dutiful wife, I tell him to fuck off to the spare room. When he ignores this and nods straight back off again, I turn over onto my other side and, quite literally, show him my arse.

Almost immediately I am wincing with pain. Do I need a new hip? Drastic, but I prefer to explore this option rather than the slightly more realistic possibility that shifting a couple of stone might help ease the pain. I toss and turn all night, rolling from side to side in an attractive fashion, looking for all the world like a large sausage in a hammock. The amount I move in bed at night far exceeds the amount I move during the day, I should wake up as thin as a fecking pencil, but the faithful flab roll is always there to greet me. On the plus side, I have lost 2 pounds this week but I think the rather large shit I had this morning might take the credit for that.

The eldest daughter is 19 tomorrow. The evening before her birth, feeling happy that my baby was fully formed and biding her time waiting to join us in the world, I had a couple of cheeky glasses of (weak) Pimm's on a very hot summer evening. When my waters broke the very next morning at 4am the smell of Pimm's was embarrassingly strong and I was surprised not to find bits of fruit, mint, cucumber and a fecking straw bobbing around.

Thus, I felt the first of many flushes of parental shame that would continue on a daily basis as I wobbled and crashed my way through parenthood. Somehow, between us, and despite us, husband and I have managed to raise two amazing young ladies, and in honour of her start in life I will raise a glass of (strong) Pimm's to my daughter tomorrow, and I will say cheers to you all too.

Scatter me happy

Tuesday July 7th 2020.

The kids and their boyfriends went to Thorpe Park yesterday
and stayed overnight. The announcement that they were
going triggered two surprising responses in me, both
highlighting the fact that I am, well and truly middle aged.
The first was to enquire how long the journey would take.
Kids were confident it was 2 and a half hours because that is
what google maps said.
I scoffed at this optimism.
My Uncle lives near Thorpe Park and I have done the
journey from Shropshire many times.
'Two and a half hours my arse' I snorted sounding, for all the
world, like my dad. 'It'll take you 3 hours on a good run'
'If you are lucky'
'It's taken me 5 hours before now'
'Better set off at the crack of dawn'
'You don't want to get caught in the rush hour traffic'
On and on and on I went. I could not stop my mouth from
spouting travel pessimism. It was like I had traffic Tourette's.
'All it takes is a minor accident and you'll be stuck on the M6
for hours, better take a flask, a spade and a blanket.'
Obviously vital equipment in July.
I found myself reaching for the AA road map and stopped
myself just in time. What the fuck? What is this madness?
Why can't I just let the kids go off and find out the hard way
that the M6 is a bitch? Why did I have to come over all
grandma about it?
The second surprising thing was what went through my
mind when I realised we would have the house to ourselves
after many, many months of lockdown. Husband and I got
in from work and sighed in ecstasy. Did we fling each other's
clothes off and start bonking on the stairs? Did husband
throw aside all the crap on the dining room table in a manly

fashion - where it miraculously landed in a neat pile on the floor - and bend me over the table cloth (clean, of course)? Did we rush upstairs and ride noisy rings round ourselves because the house was devoid of teenagers with elastic ears? No.

I walked in and nearly wept with happiness that for once I had actually come home to a house that was as clean and tidy as it had been when I left it that morning. The excitement was frantic. We dashed into the kitchen. Husband rushed to the sink and sighed with relief that it was exactly as he had left it and not crammed full of cereal bowls and half-drunk cups of tea. The worktops were gleaming, I smiled and ran my hands over them. No crumbs or drink stains. I ran to the lounge, high on anticipation. Perfect! The bliss of not having to kick my way through a mountain of trainers and re-scatter my cushions almost brought tears to my eyes! I did a little dance of joy in the living room.

This is how tragic I have become in middle age. I was so excited that I did not have to re-scatter my sofa cushions that I actually fucking danced!

Bras to bread making.

23rd September 2020

I was listening to Boris making his speech last night imposing a curfew of 10pm, and had a brief, terrifying moment where I thought he was ordering us all to stay awake until 10pm.

I expect that will be next.

He has got no chance of me complying with that rule.

9.45pm and the kids are looking at me like I have got two heads: 'Mum! You are up late'

This to the girl who, aged 17, could go all Friday night and still be at work for her Saturday job in Debenhams Lingerie department. 'Go and measure my lady's boobs in cubicle 3 please Sarah' Mrs Smith would bark, looking at me through beady, narrowed eyes and sniffing the cloud of Holsten Pils, that wafted round me, with extreme distaste.

Just what I wanted to do with a steaming hang over; lift some hairy old lady boobs up off the floor and use my entire arm span to try and get the tape measure round her.

Isn't karma a bitch? I am now the very same lady patiently waiting for a fitting and whose only goal in life is to find a decent bra that shagging well fits and lifts my tits somewhere above my belly button. In deference to my 17-year-old self, I do at least shave my nipples before being measured, though.

Last night I had a dream about getting a bread maker, so now I have truly arrived into middle age. No more raunchy, wild dreams for me. No. I have vivid dreams about making fucking bread.

I was excited when I woke up and hovered in the bleary space between dreaming and real life as, for a glorious moment, I thought I did actually have a bread maker and leapt out of bed like a child on Christmas day, only to be hammered down to earth by my bladder leaking with outrage at the sudden movement.

From bras to bread making to pissing on the bedroom floor?
Welcome to middle age.

Smash lockdown
Saturday 24th October 2020
What the heck would aliens looking down on our planet think of us at the moment?
Aliens, for me anyway, will always be the charming, darling Smash make mash creatures with their filthy laugh.
Can you imagine?
'First they put their little mask on to go in the pub' chuckle
'Then they sit down at a table and take their mask off' chuckle
'Then they put their mask on every time they stand up!' giggles
'And take it off when they sit down again!' Helpless mirth.
I was in Morrisons the other day and, unexpectedly, I coughed. It came from nowhere. A little cough that my body has produced thousands of times before, but it made me swallow my chewing gum (filthy habit) and so I began to choke. Blue faced and gasping for air I found myself apologising to everyone in a mile radius and croaking through ragged, wheezing gulps for oxygen: 'I am sorry! I am just chocking! It is not Covid!'
Finally, it passed and I lay slumped, sweating and frantically crossing my legs, hanging over my trolley and thinking that it would have been more socially acceptable if I had squatted down and twisted out a great big shit in the cheese aisle.

Now, onto the subject of clothes. Seeing as we can no longer go and try in the shops before we buy, I always order two sizes online. I hover between a 14 and a 16. Size 14 if my bloating is behaving, or size 16 if I've been on the toast and my tummy has puffed up like a bull frogs' neck.
Anyway, I tried on two pairs of the same jeans in different colours. The size 14 black denim fitted - it was a thin day.
The same size, SAME jeans in blue would not go up over my

arse. Outraged, I tried the black ones on again to make sure I had not suddenly swelled up, which is not unheard of, but no, on went the black jeans.
I checked the labels - both a size 14. I tried the blue ones again.
 'No, you lardy bitch' they said 'we will not stretch over your great flabby backside'
It is no wonder we give ourselves a hard time when this happens with clothes that are supposed to be the same size. It is a disgrace frankly. And I will outlaw it when I become Prime Minister.
Even Strictly Come Dancing got on my tits this week - fancy starting the series dancing to 'everybody's free' Are they taking the piss? Everybody is free my great hairy hole! We are all in lockdown again!
My advice? Ignore the news, grab a glass of whatever, put on a box set, cuddle the dog or cat, and try not to pluck your chin in public.
It cannot last forever, can it?

Guess Who?

8th May 2022

Had a lovely lunch today with friends and, during our conversation, one friend was trying to describe a person that we hadn't seen for years but none of us could remember her name. As we are all ladies of a certain age and our memories are not what they used to be we had to resort to asking questions such as what colour was her hair, did she wear glasses etc?

It put me in mind of the game Guess Who?

It occurred to me that there should be a guess who of menopausal women and the questions could go something like this:

Does she have a beard?
Is she sweating?
Is her face red?
Is she crying?
Is she screaming?
Is she bloated?
Does she have a moustache?
Has she got a damp gusset?
Does she look forgetful?
Has she got a dry fanny?
Is she plucking her chin?
Are her big toes hairy?
Is her growler grey?
Does she have bingo wings?
Has she got varicose veins?
Does she look anxious?
Is she saying Fuck this?
I really think somebody somewhere is missing a trick with this.

Sloppy Seconds
Monday 11th July 2022

I have been away recently to London with Mrs A and our respective husbands. When Mrs A and I go away we always have a little visit to Ann Summers, mostly just to wind our husbands up into thinking they might drop lucky on our weekend break. But also, to baffle and bewilder them with the array of vibrators at the back of the shop. The husbands look on, slightly alarmed by the thrusting, pulsing, grinding, juddering, and spinning around. If it made a cup of tea afterwards mankind would die out.

Anyway, looking in Ann Summers we came across something called a pinwheel. I literally have no idea what this is for but it looks designed to inflict some sort of pain. Mrs A took one look at this device and thought it would make a nice crimper for her apple pie. And it was not even a euphemism.
We then saw, what can only be described as yards of multicoloured rope. Again, I am not sure what the purpose is, but it looks to be some sort of skimpy outfit. I would look like I had fallen into an industrial fishing net and sex would be the last thing on anybody's mind.
Mrs A thought it would make a nice guide rope for her new awning on her camper-van.
So, we go into a sex shop and all we can come up with is apple pie crimping and tying the fucking awning down. Middle-age has arrived without much chance of having a bang.

Later that day Mrs A and I headed off to Hyde Park to see Duran Duran. I have had a crush on Roger Taylor since I was 13 years old and he is on THE LIST. The list comprises

of men that, should I accidentally fall on top of them and find myself having sex, it would not count as being unfaithful.
George Clooney is also on this list.
In my defence I fancied both long before I met my husband.
Also in my defence, my husband's list is way longer than mine and he changes it regularly. Holly Willoughby is currently number 1.

Anyway, as we were quite close to the front and I had already had a few gins, husband was feeling a bit twitchy that I might get close enough to poor Roger and do my thing. I thought he might wee on me at one point to mark his territory.

I reassured him that, in the highly unlikely event Roger Taylor should throw himself at me and beg to have a ride, I would almost certainly chicken out.
But it would make me frisky for later.
What did my gentleman husband say at the thought of a lovely, romantic night with his wife?
"I'll take sloppy seconds"
I pulled my shorts up over my flab roll and huffed off.
A lovely time was had by all, my phone ran low on battery so I could not even photograph lovely Rog because I had to leave enough charge to phone and meet my charming husband.
I told him that, alas, Roger banged only the drums.
Sloppy seconds was off the menu.

Arsehole athletics

Monday 22nd August 2022

During our recent romantic break, the mood for loving was ruined somewhat by my inability to hold in even a single fart. We were in a lovely pub crowded, of course – why is it always crowded when my bum goes off?

It was like gymnastics for the arsehole (I am imagining the BBC commentating): 'Here now is Mrs Stenton, oh and she is straight into a double trump followed by a triple puff, now she's doing the waft away followed by the spin around to see if that single bomb actually dropped something.

Watch now as she is moving gracefully across the floor doing the rare fart step - unbelievably choreographed so that a blow off is released each time a foot makes contact with the floor. Extra artistic points for the look of surprise on her face.

Timed to perfection and audible enough for the whole pub to hear.

An incredible skill!

Back into it now with the back door blast off, quite loud and lively that one, and the bend over flapper. She is finishing with the musical section; French horn long note, oh and it is a good 15 seconds long- straight into a baritone rumble, before lifting her cheek and, oh my word, the velocity in that long low tuba blow would blast off a barn door.

My word, that has got to be gold medal fluff stuff'

As we left the pub I said in a very loud voice to husband 'why can't I stop farting?

The words were just out of my mouth when a surprised and alarmed couple appeared from round the corner., giving us, quite understandably, a wide berth.

'David!' I hissed, 'why did you have to say that in my voice?'

A new low, and one I was quite proud of.

Wicked

2nd November 2022

The other night was Halloween and, in our house, something strange and spooky took place. It was dark and it was stormy, the wind howled round and the rain lashed down. Autumn had arrived. Leaves flew in and blew around the room every time we opened the door for the dog.

Dennis, the dog, who had far too much sense to go outside in such filthy weather, looked at us as if we were mad, gave us the side eye glare - the canine equivalent of flicking us the V's - promptly turned his back on us, humped a cushion and went back to his bed.

Husband looked with ill-concealed jealousy at the dog's ability to go all night without a piss, whilst I took my traumatised cushion and, dishevelled though it was, scattered it back on the sofa.

Both husband and I felt restless and unsettled. I decided to change the cushion scatter arrangement - something that would draw blood if anyone else attempted it - but still we could not settle.

The tempest got louder. The gate slammed making Dennis bark. We jumped and went to bed, watching the moon bob in and out of the storm clouds.

I wish I could sleep, I thought. Just one might…

I slept like a log. Apparently, I snored so loudly that I kept waking myself up, although I have no memory of it. I was blissfully unconscious.

My husband had a night of sheer torture during which the following were uttered, sighed, huffed, shouted, snarled, and muttered menacingly:

Please turn over

Turn over

You are lying on your back again!

Fuck's sake!

Please try and be quiet
Why can't you hear yourself?
Make a bit more noise why don't you?
I cannot believe how loud you are
I just want five minutes peace!
Why are you doing this to me?
I will just lie here and listen, shall I?
Farting as well now, are we?
It is like a jumbo jet taking off
Fecking chainsaw would make less noise
Etc.
Many fabulous hours later, I woke up from my deep
slumber, but something was different: I was feeling refreshed
and genuine shock that it was actually daylight. I felt randy. I
wanted to go the gym.
Husband looked like shite, glared at me and was grumpy.
This was a complete role reversal.
He told me what he had suffered all night.
I thought of the film freaky Friday and wondered if we had
swapped spirits.
Had I been turned into a man?
At fecking last! How marvellous! No more menopause! No
more apron flab overhang! I looked down to see if I had
balls and the family jewel hanging down.
Alas no, our metamorphosis had lasted just one night.
One night in which husband got to be an insomniac,
menopausal woman whose use of the word chainsaw was
said with relish whilst imaging it busy at work on his beloved
other half.
He got to fret and sigh and bitch and moan all night.
I got to scratch my hairy arse and sleep a beautiful sleep.
Wicked.

Rave on

20th January 2023

10 to 10 on a Friday night. Once upon a time I would have been dancing round my handbag with a vodka and coke on the go, giving it large until the small hours, not a care in the world.

Now I have done my Asda big shop, unblocked the sink, emptied my compost caddy, emptied the kitchen bin, and let the dogs out for a pee. As if that was not exciting enough, I have just taken an anti-histamine and a Nytol herbal tablet to really mix it up a bit.

Rave on ladies & gents, sleep well.

See you at 2:37 am

Miss Fire
Tuesday January 23rd 2023

A recent conversation with my husband and a contribution
from male work colleague:
Me, ranting: Why is there pee on the toilet rim? It is a tiny
hole aiming into a very big hole. How can it miss? I am
genuinely interested.
Him, not bothered: Sometimes it comes out in an
unexpected direction.
Me, incredulous: But the hole is tiny and you are pointing
downwards into a, relatively speaking, massive chasm.
Male work colleague, sticking up for his pal: Sometimes you
are half asleep and should just have a lazy wee.
Me: A lazy wee?
Men: Sitting down.
Me, sarcastic: I suppose you have to lift it up to keep it out
of the water though?
Men, sniggering: Yeah

My husband then went onto foolishly ask if my
interest/nagging was a menopause thing. Because I blame
everything on the menopause. He actually went there.
Me: As a matter of fact, the list of menopause symptoms is
longer than your arm (in fact a long arm could well be a
symptom) Flab! Itching! Fucked up memory! Stubble! Hairy
toes! Dry Fanny! Pissing myself! Farting! Hot flushes!
Insomnia! Anxiety! Anger! Sadness! Droopy eyelid! The least
you can do to improve my life is not miss fire from your
penis piss hole.
Him: You haven't got a penis so you can't comment.
Me, angry: Oh, don't worry! I'll probably grow one of those
before long.

Him: Scuttles off like a startled crab eyeing my crotch in a suspicious fashion.
I possibly should've stopped at droopy eyelid.

Sink or Slim

24th January 2023

I have recently joined, or re-joined, slimming world to try and lose this blubber buffer I have acquired since menopause. I also bounce about once a week in aqua fit.

I am afraid my mind goes to dark and wicked places at the slimming world post weigh in discussion. Although everyone in my slimming group is lovely, I clearly am not.

My mind wonders off…

Barry weighs 30 stone and has lost 7lbs this week.

'Someone please get Barry an extra chair for his other buttock. Slimmer of the week Barry! How did you do it love?'

'Well, Jean, the wife made a curry on Saturday night. She didn't have the right glasses on and put too much chilli powder in it. I'm not one for graphic details, Jean, but I could shit through the eye of a needle. Talk about a ring of fire! I was on the bog for the best part of three days. My Sandra had to put Sudocreme up me internally, if you get my drift.'

Jean: 'Perhaps we all need your Sandra's curry recipe Barry! Some of us more than others, eh Linda? Three pounds on this week love? What's gone wrong?'

'Oh Jean, I had to celebrate losing half a pound last week and so I had kebab and chips on the way home after our meeting. Then I had pizza on Friday and curry on Saturday. A nice big slimming world fry up for breakfast although I fancied sausages and black pudding with mine, plus 2 rounds of fried bread. But I did have an apple and a packet of Quavers on Monday with a cup a soup, so I thought I might have lost a bit.'

'Anna, where are you? What are you now? Six stone wet through? Another week of maintaining. That has been 403 weeks now, love, coming here every week, showing us all how to do it. What's the secret?'

'Well, Jean, I'm blessed with high metabolism, good genes and good sense. You've got to act before it is too late. I only came here in the first place because my six 6 jeans were getting a little bit tight. I cannot even look at a chip and I will not have chocolate in my house. I believe it is mind over fatter, if you'll pardon the pun. I exercise every day – it's so easy.'

Jean: 'I've got to hand it to you, Anna, you do well for a woman in her 80's'

'I'm 49!'

'Face or figure, love, face or figure. No winners whatever path you take.'

'Sarah, new girl, not hard to see which path you chose.'

'Fuck off, Jean, love'

I think I might need to give the class a miss next week and have an extra bounce around at aqua fit instead.

A serious post
5th February 2023

We all know dementia is a disease of the mind and that the
patient cannot help the way they act.
But I do not think we hear much about what it is like, as a
loved one, to reach the decision that medical intervention is
necessary. Recently I have been faced with the unpleasant
and difficult job of sorting out care for a much-loved
relative.
Why is it unpleasant? Because he does not want help and he
does not accept he has a problem.
Why is it difficult? Because we love him and do not want to
upset him.
In order to get our loved one the help he desperately needs,
an appointment was made for him to see a memory nurse. I
had to sit there and give all the reasons why I believe his
mind is becoming diseased and at the mercy of dementia. I
wonder if there is anything much more difficult than having
to state the long list of reasons, in front of my relative, as to
why I think he needs help.
You break them wide open and expose the failings and
weaknesses of their brain. You must recount personal details
about hygiene. You must explain the confusion they have
between time and distance; simple, easy things that we all
take so much for granted. You must explain that they are
confused and angered easily, stubborn, and childish, so out
of character from the kind, generous, funny person they
once were.

And you do all this with a lump in your throat. You do it feeling, utterly wretched, disloyal, and cruel. You carry on speaking with tears, rolling down your face. You carry on speaking, even though your heart aches at the sight of them, looking at you with complete indifference, like a belligerent teenager being told off. And somehow that is worse than if they shouted, denied, or even cried. Because the indifference means they do not associate that behaviour as being their own. You are talking about somebody else.

They might feel it is a conspiracy against them, because, although they may accept that they sometimes forget the odd word, they will not remember that they wear the same clothes day in day out possibly for weeks on end. They do not remember that they are not eating properly.

Your loved one will most probably resist any form of help via carers. Certainly, they will not want the memory nurse coming round and most certainly they will bitterly resent and argue against having car keys taken away.

How cruel you are to take their last little snippet of independence away from them. But you must do this. You must be the bad guy.

Because you love them.

Their minds are broken, but you break them further and expose everything you have tried so hard to cover up. If somebody we love forgets something our instinct is to prompt them and tell them what the date is, who the prime minister is or what the correct word is. If somebody wears a dirty top you remind them to put clean clothes on. If somebody looks a bit unkempt you prompt them to go and brush their hair, have a quick wash. If they forget to have breakfast you buy them groceries. Then you throw them away, rotten, and uneaten, and buy them again. If their house is dirty, you clean it. Again, and again.

It goes against everything in you to have to join all these dots up and accept that your loved one is suffering from a disease of the mind. But you do this because you love them, and maybe for a short while your loved one will acknowledge this and appreciate it.

But more likely they will blame you, they will be angry at you, and they will throw cruel accusations towards you.

And you must sit there and you have to take it, feeling guilt in every single fibre of you. Every cell burns with remorse and regret. Even though you know you have done the right thing for the right reasons, even though everybody tells you that you had to do it, I do not think you ever forget sitting there and helping destroy someone's way of life.

A way of life that was perfectly acceptable to them.

It is heartbreakingly hard.

If you too are going through similar, please know that you are not alone.

Queen Celine.
Tuesday 21st February 2023
I was looking at other menopause Facebook pages recently
and feeling a bit crap that I am not all chipper and bubbly.
I'm a moany old cow, but I quite like ranting. I'm so
outraged by the menopause that I go off like a bottle of pop.
But then I got to thinking that there is always more going on
than social media tells us, and maybe my fellow bloggers
have off days too, they just hide it better.
You might come across as a strong woman, capable and
confident, intelligent, happy and together. Or, you may look
at some of the women in your life and feel envious that they
appear to have it all. But behind every smile, there may
someone who is struggling; perhaps emotionally, mentally,
financially or physically. They might be just about coping, so
hats off to them if they can face the world with brushed hair
and a freshly waxed growler.

In the meantime, you might feel like celebrating when you
manage to find a clean pair of knickers and can actually step
into them without feeling like you have dislocated a hip.

Unconsciously, I've gone from being able to stand up, bend
over and simply pull on a pair of socks to having to sit down,
hitch my leg up as if it was in a hoist and ram the foot
vaguely towards the sock hole. When I release my leg and
stand up I always, always fart. I am slightly ashamed to admit
that I can no longer bend over and put my socks on because
my stomach gets in the way.

Putting my bra on by doing the clasp up at the back has been
out of reach for years. I can no more reach my arms behind
my back than I can fly to the moon, but when did this
happen? Without knowing or thinking about it, I have

slipped into the routine of doing the bra up at the front, sliding it round and dropping the boobs in. Obviously, great care is taken to make sure no nipple hairs get caught in the hook and eye.

You might have blank moments where you feel so fogged down you can barely be more than monosyllabic to your partner as he tries to hold a conversation with you. My husband and I did a whole journey on the M6 last week and I heard him talking but have no idea how or even if I responded. I think I occasionally grunted and mumbled, much like animal from the Muppets. I am hopeful he knows this was just because my brain had gone to the foggy place and not because I didn't want to talk to him.

And yet, when we got to our destination I bounced easily into the role of the chatty, confident, fun friend who got pissed on prosecco and sang Celine Dion into a washing up brush, truly believing it was a microphone. As well as looking like a bell end, I probably also looked like I was having the time of my life – and I was.

This menopause lark is hard, there will be tough days, and there will be really bad days. But there will also be really great days where you manage to put your nicest knickers on in one smooth, fluid, fartless movement, without stumbling and cracking you head on the chest of drawers. You will have that day where you can do your jeans up without having to squash your pubes down or trap a nipple hair in your bra, and have five whole minutes where your chin stubble is under control. You may even go two entire minutes without leaking. Little things that you once took for granted will now make you feel fecking amazing.

However, if things get really stressful, I highly recommend grabbing hold of your best friend with one hand, a (preferably clean) dish brush with the other and belting out a Queen Celine banger.
You will look like a prize knob but you will feel marvellous.

Even children get old
Wednesday 22nd February 2023

So, last night was pancake day. Eldest daughter has been
down in London and youngest daughter is away at university.
I won't lie, I wasn't going to be arsed mixing, whisking,
pouring, flipping, tossing and frying batter just for myself
and himself, when I could use the precious time to do fuck
all.
However, both daughters rocked up, lured, no doubt, by
their mother's apathy to literally give a toss, which radiated
throughout Shropshire.
But duty calls and so I shoved the menopause aside for the
evening, reached down deep and found a little bit of myself
and made pancakes for my little family. We sat together in
the kitchen eating and hatting.
I looked at my daughters and thought how exciting life is for
them. They might not feel it, one having to get out there and
work with all the twats and arseholes she will encounter and
the other studying hard for her degree, but their journey is
just beginning. We have tried to raise our beautiful girls to be
strong independent women so they can go and rule the
freaking world, but last night I found myself just wanting
time to stand still and really enjoy spending the evening
together as a family.
For a while, back in the 90's it was just me and my dog, like
the Kia-ora advert, and then along came husband. I'd love to
go back in time and whisper in the younger Sarah's foolish
ear, as she got ready for her date with the future: just take
your time and enjoy it. Treasure every second, good and bad,
painful and joyful because it is going to go so very, very
quickly.
We were soon married, I had one baby and then another, we
moved to be nearer countryside, I changed nappies and went

to playgroup, Eh-Oh! I watched fucking Teletubbies until my eyes melted, I went shopping to buy endless presents for babies at parties they would have no recollection of. I cooked mountains of fish fingers, smiley faces, chicken nuggets and baked beans in a messy kitchen for the hordes of children constantly round on a play date. I tried to hold a conversation with my husband of an evening, but his brain had shrivelled during his commute on the M6 and he could only flop in the chair and sleep, waking only to face the M6 again the next day. We had a big house, nice cars and absolutely nothing to say to each other. Enough of this shite! We took two years out to live in South West France, I don't have the words to describe how much that time meant to us, but when we returned, we started our own business so we could spend more time together and be around for our children.

Anyone who is self employed will know this is fantasy. You can never switch off.

Everything is personal.

At times it has taken more of me than I wanted to give, it has certainly robbed me of time away from my children with the awful, cruel words 'not now, mummy is working' - the working mother guilt crushed me every day for years, but we were there for sports days, assembly's, Christmas plays and harvest festivals and for that I am immeasurably grateful. Because you cannot come back and do it again.

To paraphrase my favourite song, courtesy of Fleetwood Mac time marches on and 'even children get old' and now, all of a sudden, I have two adult daughters.

One day, all too soon, they will fly the nest for good, it will be me and my husband again, and I will ignore pancake day once more in favour of shaving my bunions and plucking my big toe or whatever other delights I need to do battle with as the menopause continues to shower me with shit. But last night was lovely, and I will be forever glad for the unexpected chance to have a full, messy kitchen again.

Childbirth
24th February 2023

Yesterday I got to thinking about my first pregnancy and the birth of my eldest daughter. I should add here that we struggled to conceive and, after having a barrage of tests, I was told in a stark and bleak consultant's office, that, due to the damage undiagnosed endometriosis had wrecked, it was very unlikely I would be able to conceive naturally. This conversation still brings tears to my eyes, even after all these years. I felt hollowed out with grief. So, the last thing I want is for this to be an insensitive post to those who were unable to have children. Believe me, I know I am very, very lucky. That said, I hope you enjoy my story.

Apart from piles that felt like I was shitting out knitting needles, sometimes sideways on, I was serene and happy. Being a tidy girl, I had groomed my growler so she would look her very best, painted my nails and got my overnight bag ready and packed. On the morning before my due date, I woke up at 4.30am for a wee and my waters broke all over the carpet. Pain started coming in small waves. Having struggled with awful period pains, courtesy of the endometriosis, I decided to cope with the pain and blast on through like a warrior.

By lunchtime my knuckles were white, my vocabulary had developed some fantastically impressive swear words, beads of sweat were dripping down my face and I felt like my insides were being ripped out. I reigned curses down on my husband's penis, wishing it would blacken, shrivel up and fall off. But I felt amazingly proud of myself because, in my mind, I would by now be fully dilated and ready to push.

We went to the hospital and I expected lots of whirling around and excitement 'Well done Mrs Stenton! We can see the head" I did not expect a midwife to say: "You are 1cm along". Crushing.

On and on my labour went, through the night and into the next fecking day. Any thoughts I had of having a natural birth flew out of the window. The biggest load of old bollocks I have ever come across, is asking an unsuspecting pregnant woman to make a birth plan. What the fuck do we know? Stick your pan pipes and your cervix opening up like a flower right up your arse, and give me the drugs.

At one point, I knew, with absolute certainty, that my baby had taken a wrong turn and was coming out of my arsehole.

Finally, at 12.34pm – a whole 32 hours after my first twinge, Holly arrived looking perfect and was handed to her half dead mother.

I did not want to move, but eventually I had to go to the loo. The toilets were also equipped for wheelchair users so the mirrors were waist high. I sat on the bidet and gingerly sprayed water on my traumatised nether regions. My liver promptly slithered out of my gaping hole and drifted around in the bidet. Appalled, I pulled the emergency cord. The lovely midwife scooped up my liver, which turned out to be a massive blood clot, with two giant paper towels, and, balancing it like a blancmange, reassuringly told me that it would be sent off to pathology.

My eyes were unable to take any more horror, but, as I wobbled onto my feet and stepped towards the sink to wash my insides off my hands, I found that my fanny was level with the mirror. Huge, grey, elephant ears swung where my flaps used to be. Stretched and battered almost down to my knees. My once tidy and groomed bush looked back at me wild and wide eyed with mute terror.

And now, 21 years later, my poor old flaps look exactly the same, all the elasticity having long since left when the menopause arrived. I would cover it up with a lovely, luscious bush if I could, but a) I would have to grow it halfway down my legs and b) all I can manage these days are a few wispy grey strands with the same texture and allure as barbed wire. It is all a bit shit, really, isn't it?

Perfectly perfect
11th March 2023
Thought for the day:
I was watching The Lost City yesterday, a Sandra Bullock
film. Now I quite like Sandra Bullock she has not quite made
my lust list, but, if she plays her cards right, she could do one
day. I am sure she would be thrilled.

There is a character in this film played by. Da'Vine Joy
Randolph, and my goodness she was mesmerizing. She is big
and she is beautiful.

I felt in awe of her body confidence, I saw a beautiful, sassy,
curvy woman who was as sexy as fuck, and I say that as a
straight woman.

It made me wonder why it is that so many of us spend half
our lives on diets aspiring for the perfect body when we
might already possess one.

Why do we feel the need to look like slim film stars or
celebrities or models in magazines? Why put ourselves under
this pressure? They only represent a tiny percentage of the
population, the rest of us are just normal folk with normal
figures. Some of us are slender, some of us are tall or petite,
or large or tiny, but there is an average size for a reason; it is
because so many of us are, in fact, average.
Average height, average weight, average build. There is feck
all wrong with being like most other people on the planet.
Why are we so unkind to ourselves that we harbour
unrealistic expectations that are, frankly, unachievable?
I am horribly guilty of this. But I am trying to change.

I think we all know when we reach a size where we just do not feel comfortable in ourselves; I have put a lot of weight on over the last few years, and I started to ache all over.
I felt disgusting and unattractive and I got fed up of hating myself for it. That is why I decided to do something about it and joined Slimming World in January. However, I am confident enough to know that I do not want to lose too much weight - I just could not do it. It would mean giving up my busy lifestyle of sitting on the sofa eating crisps and drinking Gin.
I will be happy if I get to a size 14 again. My slimming world target is a lot less, and to me it is unrealistic. In order to get to a weight that ticks the BMI scale box I would have to lose 5 stone! But the BMI can shag right off.
I know my husband still fancies me, but his words fall on deaf ears; until I like myself again, I simply will not believe him. I am getting there, slowly but surely.
Maybe we need to alter our mind set instead of our body size, and accept that getting older and bigger is not a crime. If you want or need to diet for health reasons then go for it. But, instead of using celebrities as a benchmark for perfection, maybe look around at the rest of the population before you judge yourself too harshly. I think you will find you are just perfectly perfect.

13th March 2023

Middle age madness indeed

Because my (first) book is called middle age madness, Amazon has, rather hilariously, put my book in the historical section with books on the actual middle age to read alongside it.

Imagine some dusty professor searching the Middle Ages on Amazon and being faced with me in full rant about the menopause.

I am not 100% sure menopausal women folk of the Middle Ages would have been allowed to talk about ye olde hairy fanny or ye bastard hot flush. But I like to think they did:

For the love of Mary and all the saints! How hot it is in this castle solar in the middle of winter. Why are you all shivering and mewing like newborn kittens? Are not you clammy? Am I possessed of some evil fever and foul humours that will see me leave this mortal coil in my prime?

Lord knows I have acquired an abundance of body hair and could weave a blanket using mine own lady bush which has taken a life of its own and is creeping and spreading like ivy. Yet my fountain of delight has ceased to provide and is as dry as sawdust. My Lord will have to fight his way through the bush with a sword and lance only to find a dried out, shrivelled up walnut. I am forgetful, hot, and itchy as if plagued by fleas.

Have I the pox?

My Lady, ye have, as a certainty, fallen foul of the evil vapours from yonder ovaries shrivelling up. If it please you chew on a sage leaf and I counsel thee to investigate this new sorcery and witchcraft hormone replacement therapy.

So the legend goes, when your Lord and master wants to take his trouser sword from his scabbard and mount thee, you will no longer need goose grease to oil yonder fandango. You will no longer be plagued by the devil's own hot sweats and resemble a hog on the spit.

Like as not, the urge to rip thy husband's balls off and boil them in pitch will also subside.

Thy brain will not be as fluffy as unspun sheep's wool and, with the Holy mother as my witness, there will be no more hobbling to the privy chamber with thine own piss dripping under yonder tunic and chemise.

If it pleases my Lady, I urge ye to investigate with ye olde Herb Wife, so that ye may be restored to thy former gentile self. Instead of yonder raving hag before me.
Heed my words: as a surety, in years to come this period in our lives will go un-noticed because mankind will surely invent something to ease and avail us of our symptoms.

Or mayhap not…

Saturday 18th March 2023

Mother's Day.

Whether your kids are tiny, school age, teenagers, flying the nest, or have long left home; you are and always will be a mum.

From the minute you are pregnant you put yourself and your needs second to the child and this continues throughout life. You don't even know you are doing it.

You sleep with one ear open when they are babies and then again when they grow up and go off out with their mates. You will always, always worry, but you push your emotions to one side to encourage and nourish their desire for independence. From watching them roll over on a play mat, helping them hold a spoon to feed themselves, cheering them on as they learn to walk, right through to leaving them at school, riding a bike, learning to drive, having a relationship and leaving home. You are the biggest cheerleader whilst being crushed with worry and angst.

You wave them off on school trips and holidays having spent hours and hours sorting, washing, drying and packing for them.

You spend days trawling shops and the internet finding fabulous gifts for Birthdays and Christmas that you know they will appreciate.

You plan and cook lovely meals, make pack lunches, wash and dry uniforms and PE kits. You join the PTA, go to every parent's evening, assembly, nativity play and harvest festival, and act as a bouncer at the school disco. You hate the teacher that makes life hard for your child and love the ones who support and encourage your child to do their best.

You make the house look clean and nice and encourage play dates with other kids.

You bite your tongue around the little gobshites that you know your child will soon grow out of and embrace the friends you know will be for life.

You will throw yourself in front of a bus to protect your child and you would do life in jail if anybody harmed them.

You never stop caring, protecting, encouraging, loving, worrying or fighting for your child.

You put yourself and your needs second every single day. And you don't even realise it. Happy Mother's Day, you are simply awesome.

Lager vs Curry.
Monday 20th March 2023

Yesterday evening for Mother's Day, we went out as a family for a lovely Indian meal. The previous evening, I had gone to see an ELO tribute act with my husband, daughter, and friend. Husband drove and so I got stuck into the pints of lager. I have not been drinking lager for ages because of my diet, but as we were in a spit and sawdust kind of place, I felt right at home sinking the pints and getting a bonus free arm wax from any sticky surface I leant on.

My stomach began to bloat but I jiggled and I wiggled as only the drunken middle age woman can, and thought I had danced it off.

Back to last night and the Indian. Feeling like a devil after a night on the lager lash, I decided the diet could feck right off and got stuck in to a huge sharing platter. In fact, the exact words I used were: Bollocks to the diet, I am having a blowout.

Unwise, unfortunate, and scarily prophetic choice of words. As soon as I put my knife and fork together the bloat reappeared.

The bloaty, lager mass of gas met the hot spicy Indian food and the consequences were crushing for any hopes I might've had of being considered a gentile, ladylike type of mother.

My stomach gurgled ominously. My arse bubbled terrifyingly. I felt hot. I ushered my family out with all haste making it look like we hadn't paid the bill and were doing a runner.

As soon as we opened the front door to our home I began to fart. I blew myself into the living room and waited for it to stop. Alas, it did not.

My daughter's boyfriend turned up and attempted to embarrass her by reading the saucier extracts from my first diary book to her (a chapter called The Nudists). As Oscar read the story of flaps and balls hanging out in the hot Greek sun, I farted along in accompaniment, like a background brass band.

My daughter moaned an occasional feeble 'mum' and 'please no' but she was too weak with shame and mute with horror to be able to do much else.

I thought I would have to be like Big Barry, the hero of my Slimming world story of a few days ago, and have Sudocreme applied internally to put out the fire, which was raging in my rump. The curry, frankly, was much hotter coming out than it was going in.

It was an uncomfortable night, to put it mildly. Suffice to say I am now sitting rather gingerly on a cushion which has been in the fridge overnight, and I will not be going anywhere near lager, or hot curry, for quite a while.

The Nark.
Monday 27th March 2023
Because I am existing in typhoon of hormones and brain fog, I do not know if this narky mood comes round every year, every month, every week, every day or every fecking five minutes, but occasionally I get so shagged off with everything that the brain fog clears and I can see, with a clarity known only to the de-fogged menopausal brain, that I, like so many others of you, am living in a shit storm.

I survive on my nerves, 30 minutes of sleep a night and the certain knowledge that I will either piss myself, forget what I am saying, sweat buckets or fart very loudly in front of other people at some point during the day. I just accept this as normal. It is part of the carrier bag full of crap that we carry around thanks to menopause.

I know I used to be a different person, softer, gentler, and calmer. I was organised and I was efficient. I think I was nicer. Sometimes I get glimpses of old Sarah looking back at me, wide eyed with horror wondering who on earth this red faced, bearded banshee is that has taken her place. I get bloated and I get angry at absolutely nothing. I think I just like being angry. Like a bad-tempered wasp.

And Jesus, do I have wind! I have never blown off so much in my entire life as I have done these last few years. Every single day my arse goes off on a volley of farts. I have no control over it. I just wait for it to stop. Sometimes I never even notice I am doing it, much like breathing.

I can be bashing away on the keyboard at work and get the sudden urge to rub my fingers along my chin to check for any stray hair growth. Most days I wake with a Chimpanzee chin that I spend ages plucking, but there is always one bastard hair coiled under your chins that likes to unfurl in front of a customer. It evades your eyesight, waxing, plucking and hair removal cream, but will wave in the fucking wind as soon as you try to have an important conversation with somebody.

The only good thing about the nark is that I find I do not give a flying shite what anybody thinks of me and that is blisteringly refreshing. Most of the time, in menopause, I am trying to make myself smaller and keep a lid on my moods. I know I can be snappy, irritable, unpleasant and generally fucked off, but, believe it or not, I do try really hard to be nice and happy and keep the rabid, feral Sarah at bay most of the time. But the nark sets her free.

I know some people are bored of hearing about the menopause, especially those who perhaps had one hot flush, gained an ounce and once snapped at Sandra in shagging Sainsburys, but, at fecking last all the unpleasantness that so many of us have to deal with every single day is out in the open. I am so glad we are all finally talking about this and getting the word out there so that other women know they are not alone, they are not going mad and they are, in fact, normal.

Try HRT, if you can take it and if it works for you, in fact try anything you can get your hands on, but please, try talking and laughing about the menopause. Talk to your friends, and if they are not going through it, get new friends. Talk to your husband, talk to your family. Do not feel alone and do not feel ashamed. We are all in this together, keep smiling.

Why we say no
Thursday 30th March 2023
There is clearly something in the air at the moment that has sent my hormones into a tail spin.

I am having hot flushes that leave me sweating like a nun in a sex shop, my scalp is so itchy I am constantly checking for nits or fleas, which is attractive, and I am quite unable to do that most basic of human functions - shut my eyes and go to fecking sleep.

My brain and body jerk me away at 2.30am every morning. My brain is swirling in a storm of anxiety and my body is pissing sweat from every pore.
There follows the menopause Hokey Cokey: one leg in, one arm out, one flap out, one arse cheek in. Covers on, covers off. It is never ending. In fact, it is like a work out in the middle of the night in a sauna. With no escape.

All this while your beloved snores calmly and peacefully next to you. Which is just fucking infuriating and sets off the rage and pity hormone.
Rage because it is not fair that you cannot sleep and pity because nobody is around to appreciate how saintly and marvellous you are being by not waking them up to share your misery.

Instead you ride it out all night long, finally fall asleep and wake up 3 minutes later to a sprightly, bright eyed partner resplendent with morning glory nudging hopefully in your back.

I cannot speak for you all, but by this point I have all the sex drive of roadkill and feel about as desirable, so the answer is a no.
Again.
I need to clean my teeth, shower off all the sweat, shave my feral growler and everywhere else from the nose down, slather a gallon of body cream into my dry, scaly fish skin before I could even consider feeling sexy. Then I'd have to scratch about for the tube of lube and put my reading glasses on to make sure it was still in date, which is the just the height of passion and guaranteed to fan the flames of lust.

So, dear men, this is why we often say no of a morning/afternoon/evening.
We have had a shit night. We feel unattractive, we probably smell. We need the loo. Our skin feels like it is either being eaten alive by ants or shedding like a snake. Our brains are exhausted. We are exhausted. We can't remember who we are but we know we used to be quite nice. We know this is not the real us, but we cannot do much about it. We want to cry because it really is not you – it is us and we know you feel rejected which makes us sad.

But, hang in there, love us anyway, tell us we are beautiful and be patient. At some point the stars align and we have the sex surge. Lust overcomes us and we are fabulous, passionate creatures mad for a shag. We will knock down walls to get you in bed. So, save all your sexy moves for that 5-minute window. It is worth the wait.

Here comes the sun
Monday 3rd April 2023

The sun came out yesterday. Which meant an army of middle age ladies did the following:
Shaved their legs, possibly for the first time in months.
Rooted around in the bathroom cupboards for the Dove summer body glow fake tan and slapped it over freshly plucked chicken skin legs in a desperate, and ultimately vain, attempt to give them the legs of a bronzed and glowing 20 something.
If the leg has a varicose vein, then extra summer body glow was applied over and over that particular spot, in order to diminish it up with the magic cream. This resulted in a very dark splodgy patch on the leg with a varicose vein glowing brightly and proudly through it.
If you have hairy feet, and I speak from experience, you applied the fake tan, realised you had forgot to shave your feet, whipped out the razor to do the deed and were left with dark scorch marks where the hairs were.
You fake tanned your boobs, which rubbed against your upper arms spreading fake tan cream on the inside of your arms, which dried looking like a shit smear. This will not wash off and will be there for about 10 weeks. You will have to wear long sleeves all summer.
The fake tan did not take on your lower legs, but it took well on your ankles, in a very uneven, unattractive way. As if you had waded through a trough of creosote.
Exhausted after this, and crushed with disappointment that Dove summer glow does not, in fact, restore the middle age body to that of a taught, sun kissed 23 year old, the army of middle-aged women then got their uneven brown ankles and shit stained smeary arms out, sat on slightly damp outdoor cushions and had a well-earned Gin and tonic.

Am I normal?
Wednesday April 5th 2023
Whenever I write something on Facebook, I get lots of comments from ladies saying that I make them feel normal. So, I thought I would go all out and see if anyone else can make me feel better about my strange quirks.

My fanny likes chomping toilet roll. Am I the only one in possession of this unwanted skill? You can only imagine - even if you really do not want to - how spectacularly sexy I look getting my jiggle on with bits of toilet roll hanging out of me. All twirled up nicely. Like entrails.

Do you ever have a quick dust round of your bedroom with the knickers you are about to put in the wash basket? Do not get me wrong, we are not talking sexy silky expensive French fancy pants here; my pants are more Oh blah blah than Oh La La! But I catch myself doing this quick wipe around occasionally and am always surprised to look down and find my knickers in my hand rather than a duster.

Speaking of housework, do you ever kick dog hair and fluff under the rug or sofa instead of hoovering it up, simply because you cannot be bothered to get off your arse and do the cleaning? When the fluff stash is discovered, billowing out from under the sofa, like a massive cloud, usually when the door is left open and we have visitors, I am genuinely surprised by how much there is and what a dirty mare I am. I then gather up armfuls of fluff and explain in a fake shocked voice that the dog must be moulting because I only cleaned under that very settee yesterday.

Lying. It goes without saying that every new item of clothing I buy is something I have had for years or got from the charity shop or even eBay if it is discovered with the tags still on.

On my day off, I like to have a little snooze on the sofa with the hoover plugged in next to me and the feather duster in my hand, ready to leap up as soon as my other half comes home. All the better to pretend I have been busy doing jobs all day and not eating crisps while glued to the telly and the strangely addictive and hypnotic powers of Say Yes to the Dress. I then play the 'I'm too knackered to cook' card and we go to the pub for tea.

Pyjama bottoms. Even after a night of sweating, I catch myself thinking that they will last another day and convince myself that this is not only normal but makes economical and financial sense as I am saving on the washing.

Anyone else for bum hair? I have only recently accepted that my undercarriage hair has spread and branched out further. Alas, the hair is growing and climbing, like ivy, around and possibly in my bum cheeks. Hence the toilet roll bits going missing. I am disappointed as I genuinely thought I had a nice smooth bottom. It turns out that when I am trying to be sensuous, not only do I have bits of loo roll hanging out of me, I also have a hairy starfish on display. No wonder he turns the lights off.

These are some of my favourite comments in relation to this post:
Sarah: I truly get the loo roll attaching itself stealthily and then ripping the hair off with it.
Ali: I am off to change my Tena lady and check for rouge bits of bog roll up my floof.

Rose: the fecking loo roll munching drives me insane…the other day a bit dropped out of the bottom of my jeans!
Sue: OMG this has put me right off my Milky way chocolate stars!
Anne: My PJ Bottoms get the sniff test – all OK for another night?!

You sexy thing
10th April 2023

This thing keeps popping up on my Facebook time line
about Pierce Brosnan and his wife Keely.
I did not realise how much shite she has had to put up with
just because she is not some stick thin, plastic, forever young
Hollywood barbie. She has had the audacity to age naturally
and has gained weight since they got married 20 odd years
ago.
Who the feck hasn't?
Imagine living in such a shallow world that people are
actually vapid enough to ask your husband why he stays
married to you because you have gained weight?
Is he only allowed to love you if you are a size 10? Does he
not love your wit, intelligence, kindness, and passion?
Is he not allowed to love your curves and voluptuous body?
Does your husband look at you and see that you have dared
to get older or does he see laughter lines and a beautiful,
natural face with a gorgeous smile and a twinkle in your eye?
I applaud Keely for being a real woman. She looks absolutely
stunning.
You go girl, and shag that sexy husband for all he is worth,
and I will take the words I have written to you and apply
them to myself.
As should we all.
My husband is slim, fit and sexy, why do I think he would
look elsewhere because I have changed in 24 years and my
sex drive has decreased? He is a lovely man, and I do him a
disservice by thinking he would be so shallow.
Our partners adore us and we need to be better at
appreciating how fabulous we are.
It is ok to get older, fatter and saggier.

It is, in fact, normal. We are not supposed to look younger the older we get.

Having a face full of Botox, lips like a blow-up doll, a 12-year-olds body with fake boobs, no body hair, living on a lettuce leaf and having any fat sucked out of you on demand, is not normal.

It is bullshit.

Laughter lines, worry lines, saggier skin, itchy skin, hair everywhere, getting bigger, being curvier, enjoying food, enjoying drink, life experience, real love and friendship, laughter, having fun and loving life, that is what aging is all about.

And if you get to ride a sexy man as well, even if it does happen once in a blue moon, because the menopause has dried out your fanny and stolen your sex drive, I would say you are pretty much winning.

Fake it until you make it.
Tuesday 11th April 2023
Once upon a time you were a confident and capable woman. You could organise your family, excel at your job, be witty, charming and great company. You were a good, kind friend, had a fabulous sense of humour and thought life was pretty damn good. You remembered birthdays and anniversaries and always had the appropriate outfit for any occasion. You made time for family gatherings and nights out with your mates, made sure you were there for your children's assembly's, Christmas plays and harvest festivals. You even joined the fecking PTA and baked cakes.
You danced along to pop music in the kitchen as you cooked. You looked nice and made time for your husband. You were happy.
Then, just as you were feeling invincible, it all went to shit. You started to experience brain fog; that job you were so good at felt like it belonged to somebody else. You lost energy and motivation, no longer wanted to go out with friends, forgot important occasions and felt like you were wading through shit.
You got bigger, facial hair became alarming, you suffered hot sweats. You started to fart like a farm animal. Nothing fitted so you went up a size. And then another. You developed jowls that wobbled and grooves either side of your month. You looked like a cross between a bloodhound and a ventriloquist dummy. Your head was full of fluff where once witty, intelligent conversation used to live. You put your handbag in the fridge and the shopping in the wardrobe. You start saying fuck, a lot.
The more unattractive you get, the more attractive your other half becomes. This is deeply fucking annoying. You become insecure because you do not look like Davina McCall or Amanda Holden. If they can have a six pack and

still be in the menopause what the heck are you doing wrong to have a shelf of wobbly belly and a slab of arse fat? To cheer yourself up you eat a family sized bar of chocolate and a packet of crisps.

Your pubic hair is grey and sparse, but creeps down your thighs in lush abandon. Your arsehole turns hairy, along with your toes and nose. You itch so much that you check for fleas and are surprised not to find any. You feel like absolute shite and want to stay in bed all day long, yet out you get, creaking and leaking like a 90 year old, to face yet another day. You feel like someone should give you a round of applause and a fanfare but nobody appreciates how much effort it takes to get up, slap some make up on your melting face, put on clothes that you hate and face the world.

Stress and anxiety go hand in hand with the menopause: somewhere deep inside, the old you, the rational part of you, knows that the awful, gnawing, tight knot eating away at you will one day subside.

But it is still there today and will cause you yet another sleepless night as you try to wrestle with your brain and unclench the tightness in your stomach.

At night, exhausted at just surviving without making a total tit of yourself, and weary from dragging this heavy, hairy menopausal version of yourself around, you comb your hair and your moustache, slather on anti-wrinkle cream, give your armpits and knickers a sniff to see if they will do another day and climb into bed. Your partner is asleep within seconds. You wonder if he does it to piss you off. You give him the death glare. Then you lie awake next to him all night, falling asleep five minutes before the alarm goes off.

It is shite and nothing I can say will make it better, but try HRT, relaxation therapy, herbal remedies, shouting, ranting, and swearing - try what you like to make life easier. Find a group of like-minded people and talk about these changes, you will see glimpses of your old self and feel wistful. Try to appreciate that you are different, but that does not mean you are any less fabulous. Put that music on and wiggle your big old arse. Grab a drink and your friends and laugh together. Fake it until you make it. It will get better. Get some Tena Lady, keep KY Jelly handy in case you fancy some slap and tickle but your growler feels like sandpaper in the Sahara. Talk to your husband or show him this post so he knows how you feel. They may piss us off by falling asleep at the drop of a hat, scratching their bollocks and breathing loudly, but they are not mind readers and are probably quite concerned about you crying and snarling fuck off all the time.

Most of all remember you are still a confident sexy woman. You can do anything you want to do, except jump up and down unless the mop is handy.

Budapest

Thursday 13th April 2023.

A few years ago, around this time of year, my friends Julie, Val and I went to Budapest for a girlie weekend. Strolling down the street we spotted a sign that said Thai massage, great rates. Wearied by a day and night of trying to embrace the local culture by drinking so much we did not even realise the river cocktail cruise we were on had actually stopped and all the passengers disembarked, we thought a relaxing massage would be just the job.

What could be a more sophisticated, international experience than a Thai massage in Budapest?

We entered full of anticipation at the relaxing experience in front of us.

Valerie opted for the serene facial. Julie likes it tough and went for a deep tissue massage. I like to be tickled with feathers, nice and gentle so went for the full body gentle massage.

We were all in the same room, separated by thin screens. Val sat in a chair whilst a lovely young girl applied creams and lotions and potions and gently rubbed her face to make it glowing and serene. Every now and then Valerie let out a sigh of ecstasy, like a Labrador having its tummy tickled.

Julie lay on the floor, in bra and pants. Her lady was about 6 stone wet through with a nasty glint in her eye. Julie got walked on, stretched, racked, pulled, pummeled, battered, and basically tortured. She loved it. Every now and then I heard a worrying crack and she let out a little moan of pain before asking for more.

I had a very large lady who, quite understandably, spoke as much English as I do Thai. Her arms looked like enormous hams and she slammed her fists together eagerly. She looked like a prison officer about to do an internal body search. Which is basically what she did.

I had to put on a piece of string which concealed absolutely nothing. Why anybody thought sticking a shoe lace between my bum crack and up by hoof would give me any form of modesty or protection I could not say. The string rode up, my flaps flopped over each side. I felt like I was sitting astride a washing line.
My prison officer got to work with my gentle massage which was not, in fact, gentle. She kneaded by backside like it was day old dough, working those knuckles down deep and firm, making my shoelace clad bottom clench in horror. She went everywhere. I was mute with horror and closed my eyes willing my mind to float away. Julie was being racked, Val sounded like she was having an orgasm and I was dangerously close to becoming a glove puppet.

Naturally, being British, I thanked her afterwards for giving me a gynecological examination instead of the gentle massage I had paid for, and we went on our merry way. Val looking like she had had the best sex of her life, Julie looking like she was on stilts and me unable to sit down for 24 hours afterwards.

But it was an experience we still talk and laugh about five years later, although my hand goes instinctively to my bottom, and I give an involuntarily wince every time the subject is raised.

I know the menopause makes us feel shitty, but here is to our fabulous friends who carry us through, keep us laughing and are just there to get through life with us.
We women really are awesome creatures.

Taste of Paradise
Monday 17th April 2023

This is an unusually sexy post for a Monday. But the starts
have aligned and decreed that I will be given the horn today.
Perhaps I had better explain.
I came to work full of the usually Monday joys with a face
like a slapped arse. I parked myself next to my colleague Paul
"I'm not buying your book when I sit next to the live show
every fucking day" when our friendly fire was disturbed by
the electricity board chopping up the High Street with very
loud machinery.
It is so noisy we are trying to communicate by sign language,
but we only know the V's, the finger, wanker and knob head,
so our conversation is quite restricted.
In despair, I went up to the post office and, on the way saw
one of the workers, who said 'Hello pet' and called me a
bonny wee lass. I do not think I have ever been called a
bonny wee lass before.
I was so surprised that I stopped and said hello back, only to
get looked up and down in manner that reminded me of a
dog eyeing up a juicy pork chop. He was so subtle he may as
well of dropped his pants and asked me if I fancied a go on
his hairy cock.
I walked quickly on, partly because I was tempted to knee
him in the balls for perving, but mostly because my vanity
was screeching at me to move before Mr Subtle realised that
the pork chop was perhaps not as fresh and juicy as he might
have thought, and also likely had a bit of hair stuck on it.

Back to the office and the noise escalated. Just when it
became unbearable the office started to judder and shake as
they started using another machine. This provided a
sensation that was not unpleasant.

My seat vibrated in a way that people would pay good money for. It got a bit faster. It got a lot nicer.

This was better than anything you might find in Ann Summers and put a smile on my miserable Monday morning face.

I even thought about nipping over the chemist and buying some feminine lubrication products in case I still feel tingly later on, at home.

Husband came and stood by my desk and I had a conversation with him whilst eye level with his denim clad groin. I stared at it with an intensity that would make Mr Subtle die of embarrassment.

Also today, whilst my chair was merrily vibrating, a very kind reader of my Facebook page suggested to me that those of us with dry foo foo's can use coconut oil instead of expensive tubes of lube. Alas and alack, my beloved dislikes coconut and would not go near a Bounty bar flavoured growler. No taste of paradise for him!

Warrior

Wednesday 19th April 2023

I find it so very sad that some of us get to a certain age and no longer like ourselves very much. I have been through it myself – I was ashamed of my body, felt blah and just could not be arsed to do anything.

I fell into a depression. I am not saying that was down to me not getting the grind on with my man; in my view it was 100% to do with the menopause or peri-menopause and how it made me feel.

If I washed my hair, it was a good day. I just did not feel worth that small, normal act of basic personal hygiene.

You think that everybody will notice the crisis happening to you, but the truth is they do not. You get pretty good at coping and plodding on. Going through life like a robot, numb to pretty much any feeling. You smile when you need to smile, give a half-hearted laugh if it is required, feign interest, and just exist, feeling bleak and dark and very, very lonely.

I have been there and I know it is a tough place to crawl out of. I used to look in the mirror at my dead eyes and wonder where I had gone. I just could not claw my way back and, if I had not been so empty inside, I would have felt my heart break for me.

If you feel at all down and have lost interest in all or any aspects of your life, please open your mouth and talk. Tell your partner, tell your friends, tell your doctor, tell anybody who will listen and get the help that you deserve. And you do deserve it. We are only here once and being a woman is hard enough without having to drag the weight of depression around with you.

The outrage is that so many of the symptoms that lead us middle aged ladies to feel depressed, are caused by the onset of the menopause. I still do not think we are all taken seriously enough when we see our GP and try to ask for help. It takes courage to sit opposite someone and open up to them.

You are making yourself vulnerable and far too many of us come away having being made to feel like we have wasted time and are not worth the effort of further investigation. Fuck that, frankly. It is about time we were listened to and given proper help. Just because we can just about cope, does not mean we should have to.

This is half the population I am talking about who have been given the shitty end of the stick. You know your body and yourself better than anybody. You are worth the fight. Thankfully my husband did notice I was struggling and made me see the GP who put me on anti-depressants. I was on them for 4 years. During that time, I started writing on Facebook, mainly because I could not find anything or anybody I could identify with

Somewhere, somehow, as I wrote my diary, my sense of humour came back and I found I could make this sea of shit a fun place to be, surrounded by other like-minded women who had been silently screaming as they tried to cope. I am also so proud that men follow this page to see what life is like for their wives or partners (shit, since you ask).

So, keep going ladies and find something that makes you feel like you. Even if it is sitting on the sofa eating chip butties and plucking your chin hair. Which is my happy place.

I have good days, I have bad days, but that is just life. I have learnt to love and respect myself. I am bigger, I am hairy, I sometimes smell quite nasty. I am quick tempered, I have spectacular road rage and an impressive vocabulary of swear words, I can fart the alphabet out of both holes, I am itchy, I cannot remember shit and I am tired. But I am a menopausal, middle-aged woman and that makes me a warrior.

20th April 2023
Love Honey
Not that I am sex mad or anything but I keep thinking of those of you who have lost the desire and feel bad about it, those of you who want sex but think the old girl has healed up and those of you whose husbands would not look up from the telly even if you started twirling nipple tassels and poured a pint of beer with your hoof.

A few years ago, I made a purchase from Ann Summers (they are not sponsoring this by the way, although they fecking well should be!)
It is NOT a big scary pulsing, pumping, grinding vibrator that needs powering by the national grid and will twirl you around like a carousel.
No. This is - not sure I can say this delicately - for external use.
I am no sex therapist, God knows what the right advice is, but this put a smile on my face and gave me all the lovely feelings.
Your man can be there or you can fly solo.
But treat yourself. It is marvellous. Get it out of the box and get on it.
You can thank me later, there are others at different prices, but this one is worth every last penny.
It is called The Moregasm – and is marvellous.

Favourite comments:
Eileen: Check out LoveHoney.co.uk The judge at my divorce hearing thought I was a beekeeper reading my bank statements!
Annette: I had a plumber in doing some work in one of my airing cupboards, not realising he needed access I moved

some black bin bags. One of them started to buzz…he never did come back!

Jill: I have a box in my bottom drawer with a note to my kids stuck to the top saying – DO NOT OPEN, chuck this in the bin. Inside there is a note saying 'Don't say I didn't warn you!'

Linda: I think the Ann Summers website is about to crash.

Deb: Wow! At that price it better take me out to dinner first!

Hazel: I had a pink clitoris toy with feathery bits on it which fitted over your vulva…imagine my horror when my 5-year-old came downstairs with her new 'gum massager' that she had found!

Anonymous message: Just had to say that my hubby treated me to the Moregasm for my birthday...OH MY GOD!!!!!! Thank you, thank you thank you!

Head and Shoulders
Sunday 30th April 2023
Apparently, we have had the coldest April since 1986. In
fact, it has been so cold and so rainy that I have refused to
shave my growler because:
a) there is no chance of wearing shorts in this weather, (be in
no doubt, I need to trim it even for the longest shorts).
b) it is an extra layer of fluff to keep me warm
c) I cannot be arsed.
But on Friday, in the shower, even I realised it may have got
out of hand. Without thinking I actually used Head and
Shoulders shampoo on my foo foo because I was worried
about it getting dandruff.
Oh dear. Wax on order, pronto

Menoshit vs Marriage
Tuesday 2nd May 2023
I have recently had the most enormous poo I think I have
every done. I am not sure if this is the menopause or not, I
mean God knows everything else has gone to pot with my
head and body, so why not let my ability to have a crap join
in too?

The menopause is a battle ground, we all know that, and we
fight on as best we can, I sometimes forget how many things
about me have changed. And so it is that every now and then
along comes a shite so massive and eye watering I almost
expect a midwife to appear encouraging me to push, wrap it
in a towel and stick a bonnet on its head.
The last time I had this was a few years ago, when Sky man
was round installing boxes and drilling holes for cables. I had
to wait for him to start drilling through our, mercifully thick,
stone walls to drown out the noise of my grunts and groans.
I was literally on the loo for 45 minutes, I cannot imagine
what he thought I was doing in there all that time, but I came
out walking like John Wayne after a year on horseback.
This time round I dived on the loo in front of an outraged
husband, who was in the shower. I explained that I only
wanted a quick wee and thought I would admire the view of
his bum whilst I tinkled away.
He shrugged reluctantly. No harm no foul.
Alas, out of nowhere my bowling ball mega menoshit
arrived. My husband was by now in the middle of his shower
and could not escape. He had to endure the full show.
I went to another realm of pain and shame. I know I was red
faced and sweating. I pushed up on my hands to try and
levitate off the loo and let gravity have a go, when that didn't
work, I crouched down and squeezed. Up and down I went
for a long time and I remember thinking I had not had to

push this hard since a human head came out of me. I was convinced for some time afterwards that I had ripped myself a new arsehole.

But eventually the deed was done. Naturally, my humiliation was incomplete, because the beastly thing refused to flush away and almost blocked the loo. Walking with my legs splayed as far apart as I could get them, and clutching onto to what was left of my shredded bum hole, I went to find my husband who had escaped shower hell and was in the bedroom. His morning, already faring lower than a snake's belly after my toilet gymnastics, took yet another downturn when he had to unblock the loo to the sound of me retching and gagging in the background.

By mutual agreement, we have decided for the sake of our marriage to never to speak of this event, at least until the next time the menoshit pays me a visit.

Things that make women happy
Wednesday 3rd May 2023
Scatter cushions placed in very specific positions on the sofa
scatter pillows plumped up and crease free on the bed
Throws placed with strategic accuracy to the millimeter, to
look like they have been casually flung over the back of the
sofa
Throws placed with painstaking precision at a jaunty angle
across the bed to look carefree and rustic
Setting the table for Christmas dinner 3 weeks before
Christmas
Hanging out the washing neatly to show off all the nice
sheets and pillow cases to the neighbours, whilst hiding the
grotty knickers.
Scented candles
Baskets for displaying how many toilet rolls you have left
Freshly washed and fluffy towels for guests
Lovely sparking taps and sink
Clean, freshly bleached toilet
Putting the furniture and lovely cushions outside ready for
summer sun
A fully stocked fridge overflowing with loads of food and
drink

Things that piss women off:
People sitting on the sofa and disturbing the cushion
placement.
Somebody sleeping in the bed and messing with the display
pillows
Somebody feeling cold and using the casually flung display
throws to keep warm
People thinking they can sit down at the ready-for-Christmas
dinner table and use the best plates before Christmas day
Interfering with the washing by hanging it all wrong and

displaying grotty grey knickers to neighbours
Lighting the scented candles when no visitors are expected
Using the toilet rolls in the display basket
The freshly washed and fluffy guest towels being used. Even
if it the guests using them.
Toothpaste spit and a curly hair in the gleaming sink 30
seconds after you have cleaned it
People actually using the clean, freshly bleached toiler
The fecking British weather pissing down on the lovely
outdoor cushions.
A plague of locusts going through the fridge five minutes
after you have filled it.

More Bognor than Barbados
Wednesday 10th May 2023

God love us, but the menopause drags on and on, doesn't it?
I've been at this for 4 years already and get the feeling I have
barely scratched the surface, yet I think I have had pretty
much every symptom going.
Itchy skin – like I have fleas or nits.
Hairy chin/nose/upper lip/nipples/toes/even the tops of
my fecking feet
Disappearing eyebrows except for one insane long one
which unfurls like a wasp antenna
Disappearing growler hair – why does it need to turn into
wire and leave vast bald patches?
Saggy flaps
Saggy arse
Saggy boobs
Saggy jowls
Saggy upper arms
Depression – hardly surprising
Zero pelvic floor muscles – sneezing, coughing, and God
forbid, jumping means I piss myself.
Zero back door muscles – bending over, standing up, even
fecking walking releases a volley of farts
Brain fog which leads to confusion, anxiety, stress and
embarrassment.
Insomnia, just when I want to switch my brain off it springs
into life and twirls and whirls all night long.
Hot flushes – just when you finally do fall asleep you are
woken abruptly because you are drowning in your own
sweat.
Dry fandango – like a drought in a desert.
Loss of sex drive – no wonder when you feel as attractive
and desirable as a sexual disease.

Taking ages to orgasm - and even then, your destination is more Bognor than Barbados. And we deserve Barbados.

Mood swings – I have never felt so angry at absolutely nothing, but that is the menopause.

Weight gain – because we have not got enough going on to make us feel shitty.

Apathy – fuck it, I'm fat anyway so why not eat a bag of crisps?

Confidence – swings from being lower than a snake's belly to feeling I can stick two fingers up to the world and saunter about not giving a shite what people think.

So, over the years I have tried to come up with ways to make this shit trip more bearable. First and foremost, keep smiling and laughing at this fecking outrage, most of us are going through it so grab a glass of Gin and get together with your friends. Mention the unmentionable and have a giggle together.

Treat yourself to a lovely massage or facial

Buy clothes that fit and flatter instead of giving you bingo wings and a slab of belly fat; who cares if you have to go up a size? Elastic was invented for a reason.

Keep shaving/waxing/plucking, or get it lasered off. Or take your glasses off so that you cannot see the hair. Alternatively, just go feral, who is to care?

Wear piss pants or piss pads – it is not worth the risk to go commando, you'll be dripping like a faulty tap.

Buy a sexy nightie that covers all the wobbly bits but shows off the cleavage or your legs – if your partner sees boob or a shapely leg, he won't notice anything else.

Get yourself a sex aid from Ann Summers or Love Honey and a tube of lube.

Book a few nights away, somewhere with a hot tub and go relax with a bottle of prosecco. Leave Bognor behind and get yourself to Barbados courtesy of Ann Summers airways.

Draw your eyebrows back on with eyeshadow – not blue, obviously.

Make the best of what you have got, have a hair cut, get some new make up, buy a new bra.

Accept that you are changing and you are different and that this is a challenging time in your life and it is OK not to feel OK about it.

Try herbal supplements, sleeping aids, HRT whatever floats your boat.

Keep talking about it – nobody knows how shit you feel unless you tell them.

Give in and have a cry or a scream - you have got so damn good at coping with everything for such a long time that it really is OK to let some of the spinning plates drop and put yourself first.

We have raised our kids, run a house, held down a job and very often played second fiddle to everyone else's needs. The menopause might be shit, but this is our time to reach out and say 'me first.' You deserve it.

Shit Happens
Tuesday 16th May 2023
Saturday morning started fantastically well with the immortal words, shouted mournfully up the stairs: 'David, I've just shit myself a bit.'

I had been feeling a bit off all night with crampy pains, finally fell in to a deep sleep around 4am and was abruptly woken up at 7am by loud gurgling from my tummy. I was still sleepy and vaguely and foolishly tried to ignore it. My tummy gave a spasm of warning. This was followed by the urgent, eye-popping realisation that I no longer possess the ability to hold in any form of toilet activity. I flew out of bed, hand on my pyjama clad bum, dashed to the En-suite to find my husband already in situ and in no hurry to move off.

This was dire, I now had to dash down the stairs, over the spaniel stair gate and launch myself at the downstairs loo. Do not imagine for one minute that I hurdle over the stair gate like Colin Jackson, I carefully hoist one leg over it, gripping onto the gate as if I were dangling off the edge of a mountain rather than being one step up from the floor, and then heft the other leg over, as if I were lifting a giant ham. Alas, the spaniel stair gate was a leap too far for the middle-aged slack arse hole and, somewhere astride the gate, my sphincter gave way.

Spaniel and Labrador, previously eager to greet their mummy, backed off whining. I waddled with absolutely no dignity at all, whining a fair bit myself, to the loo and stayed there until David came to the rescue.

Later that day, unleashing the middle age women mindset of 'thou shall not miss a party when there is free booze' I made myself recover enough to dress up in red white and blue and go to a friend's Eurovision party on Saturday night. In easily the single most brave and stupid act of my adult life, I even wore white jeans and prayed there would be chocolate mousse so I could at least say I had accidently sat in some, should the worse happen. Again.

Halfway through a bottle of Pimm's, my tummy groaned and rumbled once more, alas, there was no chocolate mousse to take the blame, although there was a rather lovely Tiramisu, and so I retreated home and was tucked up in bed by 10pm. I am better now although I still don't dare fart too far away from the loo, just in case. Naturally, as farting happens as often as blinking, this means I am up and down every five minutes.

When I previously wrote on Facebook about poo, I got a snooty reply telling me that I was disgusting for talking about this subject to try and get a laugh. Here is my reply: These things happen as you get older, I have ulcerative colitis (although very mildly, thankfully) and my arsehole resembles an open trap door. Accidents can and do happen, especially if there is a tummy bug about. It is important to find the lighter side and to be able to laugh at the absurdity of it all. I am not going to crawl away burning with shame. I hope that by addressing these issues other women can think it is OK to laugh and to know that they are not alone with whatever they are having to carry around. If this subject is not your cup of tea, move along and wait for something more agreeable to pop up on your timeline. But please, do not try to make me out to be wrong, vile, or vulgar for bringing these subjects out in to the open.
Shit happens, change your pyjamas, and get over it.

The Manopause
28th May 2023
This afternoon I watched a sad video with my daughter. We both cried. I had eaten pickled onions and sobbed so loudly, that, much to my surprise, I farted.
Loudly.
I was outraged by this lack of control. Is this another string to my menopause bow; is my arse so slack I cannot even have a good old cry without letting rip?
To cheer me up, my husband fished out the fan and set it up in our room. At times like this I find him extremely attractive.
Alas, he ruined the moment and went on to say that he also needed the fan due to the Manopause.
What are the symptoms that my beloved is experiencing?
Does he fart without warning, shit boulders, sweat, cry, leak, have dry balls, ache, forget and feel like he is going round the bend?
Oh no, the Manopause makes him feel horny in the morning.
That's it.
I rolled my eyes and leant over to turn the fan on.
I farted, of course.

Acceptance
Wednesday May 31st 2023

And so, another summer is nearly upon us, and once again I
am bigger than I would like to be, and, once again, I have
done feck all to facilitate any real change.

But then I asked myself why I wanted to change anyway, and
the answer is that there is so much pressure to look good. It
is all around us: in the media, on holiday advertisements, on
magazine covers, on the TV. You never see a middle-aged
woman, stuffed into a swimming costume as tight as a
sausage skin with hairy bits of groin or armpit bursting out
from the elastic, swigging a cocktail at a beach bar on the
holiday adverts, do you? But that is what most woman on a
beach look like. And we are the ones most likely to organise
the fecking holiday! Note to TUI, Jet 2 etc – we are not all
nubile, nympho 25-year-olds with a washboard stomach and
a tidy, tight fanny. Sometimes the saddle bags flop out of the
saddle.

So, this year, instead of giving myself a kicking for not being
the slim, toned, honey coloured goddess of my imagination –
so perfect that a pubic hair would not dare pop its head up
anywhere near my bald little biff – I am going to try
acceptance.

Acceptance that I am nearly 52, and I am the shape and size
I am because I love food and drink as much as I hate
exercise. I am a size 16. I do not like my muffin top fanny
roll, and I'm not keen on my legs, but mostly I have curves
in all the right places. I am all for women doing whatever
they want to do to look as good as they can, but I do despair,
on behalf of the rest of us, that some of the celebrities go

too far. I see a perfect, glowing, glossy, tiny woman on TV, the same age or older than me and think I must be doing the menopause wrong because I am a little bit fat with a five o'clock shadow and can fart the national anthem.

But I do not want to look like a 12-year-old. I am all woman. My boobs are good. In fact, they are fabulous. Nice big bouncy boobs! You do not get those on a barbie doll body full of silicone

I have got creases and wrinkles, grooves, and frown lines. I have got hair growing in places that is frankly wrong and baffling – why exactly do I need a hairy arsehole? My eyesight has gone to shite and my memory is awful. I am prone to leaking piss wherever I go, and shit myself last week climbing over a stair gate.

But feck it all, I am here, and I am fit and well. This body and brain have been through an awful lot and have lived to tell the tale. I think I need to be a bit kinder to them.

The Dentist
Saturday June 3rd 2023
Yesterday I went to the dentist to have three composite
fillings put in near my guns to try to stop them receding any
further and leave me looking like a horse. All were on the
top front teeth, one in the middle, one to the right and one
to the left.

Our dentist is quite dishy and fit. Especially since he has
started going grey and wearing a beard.
This never usually crosses my mind except to be glad we
now have him rather than the mono brow, scowling,
chainsaw loving Eastern European woman butcher we used
to have.

I am not a fan of going. I always lie about flossing my teeth.
We both know I am lying but I do it anyway. I do not like
the thing that sucks your saliva out. I do not really like any of
it.

But teeth are important, so I go anyway and having an
attractive dentist makes it a little bit more bearable.

There he was looking all sexy and knowledgeable in his
scrubs, a bit hot and bothered because he had just had a
difficult conversation with someone.
He was brooding and moody.
Like Mr Darcy, in scrubs and trainers.
Masculine energy was in the room, despite being very happily
married to a living saint, my vanity antenna sprang into
action: 'hot man alert! Breathe the fuck in!'

I lay in the chair which was fully reclined and lowered. I obligingly opened my mouth and the dentist got to work. Front tooth gum area first. Then the right side, so I had to turn my face to the left.

Then he needed to work on the other side, so I had to turn my wide-open mouth to the right, where he was sitting astride his stool.

My gaping gob was now just inches from his groin.

I told myself not to think it.

A hot flush crept over me, that, for once, was absolutely nothing to do with the menopause.

I pleaded with myself not to go there.

I squeezed my eyes shut and tried to think about putting the bins out.

Nonetheless, the saliva sucker had to go up a gear thanks to an excess of drool.

Shovel my shit and call me Sally
Wednesday 7th June 2023
I have just read my 'Sarah' post which I wrote in January
2018 and was the start of this page taking off. I have
included it right at the start of my first book, for anyone who
wants a reminder. If you had told me five years ago that I
would still be writing about the enormous shit that the
menopause keeps twisting out in my direction I think I
would have just stared back at you in appalled shock.
But here I am; older, and wiser now, to the ups and downs
of Madame menopause.
I cannot do a lot about the exodus of hormones so I would
rather try and laugh my way through it instead of crying.
I am fucked off 85% of the time, and for no particular
reason. I have learnt to accept this and quite enjoy being full
of rage. I was always quite nice and a people pleaser before
my hormones crashed out of my pelvic floor. Now, if
someone does not like me, well shovel my shit and call me
sally – I genuinely do not care unless someone is rude. Then
I get sparky.
My morning routine is now as follows: have a wee and a
massive meno shit, pluck my chin, shave the stubborn bristle
that I can reach with tweezers, lift my boobs up to see how
much lower they have gone, squeeze my flab roll to see if it
has gone down after my meno poo, slather my face with
moisturiser to stop it drying out like a prune, stick some
make up on, paint on my eyebrows with brown eyeshadow
as they appear to have suddenly disappeared, sniff my pants
to see if the piss pad has been a suitable buffer and the pants
will do another day, get dressed and face the world.
I spend most of the day at work wondering what I was just
in the middle of doing or saying before my brain was
enveloped in a wave of fog, and convincing myself that
Quavers do not count as food because they are cheese

flavoured air, and a Fruit and Nut chocolate bar is basically a vegetable.

In the evening I go home, get changed into pyjama's at 6pm and wonder how the 'fro below has sprouted so much in the 24 hours since I last looked at it. Spend a few minutes hacking vaguely away at it with scissors, but avoid the saggy flaps at all costs. They can stay hairy. Look in the mirror expecting a nice tight, pretty fanny. Alas, my foo foo resembles an old bald man with a straggly goatee.

Spend the evening watching crap on telly and moaning about it before nodding off at 9pm. Fart my way upstairs to bed, leave my make up on because who can be bothered to wipe it all off, get in bed and am suddenly completely unable to sleep. Fan on, book open, mind a whirling mass of all the things I was supposed to remember to do earlier that day. Lie on one side and my knee aches, lie on the other side and my hip starts hurting. Lie on my back and my boobs flop under each armpit in a pool of sweat. Huff and puff and say fuck a lot. Husband falls asleep instantly which enrages me. Every day is the same and we all cope in our own different ways. I try to avoid sneezing, I talk to my husband about how I am feeling, even he really does not want to know and that includes my explaining about my fluctuating sex drive. My husband knows that if I am in the mood, he better get his shit together and lube up because the window is liable to slam shut any second.

If you are just starting on this journey and are wondering where on earth you have gone, then I have been there and can tell you that you do slowly, get a bit of yourself back again. Laughter is the best medicine, remember it is not just happening to you it happens to most women of a certain age, so talk, talk, and talk some more.

That lovely, slim, toned body will vanish and you will look like you have eaten your old self, but you will learn to say fuck it and wear clothes that suit you instead of trying to squeeze into jeans that refuse to do up.

And ignore the media. The celebrities have teams of people around them and pots of money to look unreal, frankly. Nobody has a six pack unless it is of crisps.

It has been 5 years of living in a sea of shit, but, instead of floundering neck deep, I think I am now surfing on the sea and, sometimes, I even enjoy the ride.

Fuck it all til Friday
Thursday 8th June 2023

I have just met the nemesis of all middle-aged women…the
changing room mirror. I normally only look at myself chest
up and can therefore be in ignorant bliss of the spread
below, but the changing room has mirrors placed at all angles
so I get to see the back, front and side view.

I won't lie, it was not pretty. I am still overweight despite
losing over a stone, but I will never have a lithe, toned slim
body again. I know this because I like food and booze too
much and I dislike exercise.

In the changing room I was relaxed and my belly looked like
it did when I was nine months pregnant, I had a shelf of
back fat and looked like I had gone to seed. The old me
would have been horrified and disappointed. But the 51-
year-old me was OK. I shrugged it off and thought bollocks
to it.

Unless I can pop a magic pill to make me wake up as a size
10, I will always flinch a bit when I catch an unexpected sight
of me from the side or the back. But fuck it all 'til Friday,
this is who I am and I am starting to be more accepting of
that. I would not take back all the lovely meals I have eaten,
or even the lazy packets of crisps I have scoffed on the sofa.
I would not undrink all the delicious cocktails I have
enjoyed, or the pints of larger I have drunk with friends by
the river on a sunny day.

I have enjoyed every single mouthful and my body is the
result. It looks OK with clothes on and my husband is happy
enough with the clothes off so who am I to complain? I

think I am starting to forgive myself for getting older and fatter and it is empowering.

A smile, a laugh and a fun personality are more important than having a perfect body. I know I would rather be out with a group of girls who enjoy their food and like a good time instead of being with somebody who picks at a salad and a low-calorie tonic water for fear of putting on a pound. I can shit out a pound, it is not worth worrying over.

I am curvy, and yes, a little bit fat. But I am the girl you want to take out for a nice long lunch and have a giggle with. I will just finish by saying look at yourself as others do and be kinder you yourself. You are a gorgeous creature.

Queens
20th June 2023
What we think of ourselves:
Fat with Belly overhang
Hairy as fuck
No sex drive or Nympho urges
Sweaty
Raging
Forgetful
Resting bitch face
Unable to give a feck
Ugly
*

What our partners think:
Lovely curves
Spends a lot of time shaving
Sex goddess
Glowing
Always been a bit snappy
Happens to everyone
Lovely smile
Confident
Gorgeous

We are beautiful, stunning, amazing women neck deep in menopause shit!
We are still in there somewhere and maybe we need to see ourselves as others do instead of comparing ourselves to celebrities and finding ourselves lacking.
Fabulous, powerful Queens, with flab, stubble and a dry fanny. We are real women, and we are fantastic.
Love yourself a little bit more today, see yourself as others do. Hold your head high and your bum cheeks together to stop that fart escaping in public.

Chimpanzee chest.

Thursday 22hd June 2023

I am a middle-aged woman fighting my way through the changes during this strange time in my life.

I do not always get it right. I get cross and narky more often than I used to.

But then I am dismayed at the changes to my body and mind. I do not enjoy shaving my nipples, or my thighs. And why exactly do I need a moustache and chin hair at the age of 51? I have managed perfectly well without either, until now. It is not like I suddenly feel the cold or anything because I am always so fecking hot!

I do not like my chunky legs with the delightful varicose vein snaking its way down my calf.

I cannot stand the insomnia, and the memory fog. I feel dopey and dumb where once I was intelligent and capable.

I know the old Sarah is still in there somewhere, trying to claw her way back, albeit under an extra 3 stone and a beard. The menopause has shit on me, but I refuse to be beaten.

I wear a piss pad every day because I pee myself when I sneeze, jump, trip over or laugh.

And I like to laugh. I like to laugh a lot, so I leak. So what? It is not the end of the world. If I sneeze too violently, I must dash off and change my pad, or upgrade to the big sexy nappy knickers, on the occasions where the pad throws up its wings and admits defeat.

It happens to a lot of women and it is nothing to be ashamed of.

I fart so often that I barely notice I am doing it anymore. My bum cheeks flap so much they help keep me a bit cooler.

I wear shorts because fuck it, they are my legs and if you do not like them then look away.

I shave my nipples because I do not want a chimpanzee chest.
I pluck my chin and wax my moustache because I am too vain to walk around looking like a nanny goat.
My sex drive packs up and leaves town for months, and then returns with a vengeance for about 25 minutes.
(I shave my thighs on these occasions, otherwise my hairy husband and I will be stuck together like Velcro, and it is far too hot for that).
Fight the good fight, do what you can, take whatever drugs work for you, but remember - you are not alone.
Laugh, leak, shave, pluck, say fuck more than you used to.
But enjoy life and keep laughing.

Beach Life part one
Sunday, 25th June 2023
Arcachon, France
Today is the last day of our holiday. I am sitting on the
beach, people watching.
I see ladies who are self-conscious about their bodies and
hide away in baggy cotton cover ups, right until the very last
minute before they brave the walk to the sea.
I see larger ladies taking shelter under a parasol because they
do not feel confident enough wearing swimwear, but they
want to be part of the beach visit nonetheless, and spend this
time with their families.
The lady in front of me is sitting in a deckchair, under her
umbrella, wearing a dress that covers her body, watching her
family frolic in the surf.
She was very cautious about putting her weight on the flimsy
deckchair and my heart aches for her.
Her family are trying to encourage her to join them but she is
using the excuse of guarding the bags as a reason not to strip
off, throw caution to the wind and plunge in the ocean.
I think we have all been this lady at some time or another. It
is a story that is repeated on every beach on every holiday.
I also see men looking at their partners in admiration, eyeing
up their curves appreciatively when the shirt or sarong is
finally discarded.
The women do not notice this.
They are in too much of a hurry to hide beneath the waves.
There are gorgeous young, lithe bodies everywhere, looking
effortlessly sexy in their swimwear. Male and female.
Yet the older, larger men do not hide under clothing. It is
always the women.
We are too hard on ourselves. Hiding our aging bodies away.
The media gives us images of perfection and it is unrealistic,
unachievable, and damaging. 50-year-old bodies do not look

20 years old unless serious work or extreme lifestyle changes have taken place.

There is always going to be someone slimmer and younger than you. Usually, the fuckers sit right next to you, doubling the inadequacy. But take a look around, there is also always someone older and bigger than you.

However, there is only one of you.

The camera and the mirror may not like you anymore.

But your husband or partner loves you.

Your family love you.

Your friends love you.

In 30 years' time the nubile lithe bodies will be older, just like us.

My body is far from perfect, if magazine covers are what we judge perfection on.

But, at the age of 51, after two children, and a life spent eating crisps, drinking gin, and laughing, it is perfect to me.

I am going to dance in the surf, wobbly thighs, bingo wings and all.

I hope I can encourage the lady in front of me to fling her dress off and do the same.

Favourite comments:

Christine: I'm 72 today and in Zante. I don't give a flying fuck what anyone thinks so whip my bikini top off as soon as I hit the sunbed! If anyone is offended by my brown boobies, then look away now!

Darren: Us gay guys have the same worries too as heaven forbid we don't have the six pack and pec chest that all the 20+ generation sport by spending 8 million years in the gym. We all get older and less in shape, but I know one thing; if I had a choice between cuddling a guy with a six pack or cuddling a dad bod with curves, I'm taking the dad bod!

Beach Life part two.
Tuesday 27th June 2023

(This entry was written after I had shown a picture of me dancing in the surf on holiday – I had a swimming costume on, thankfully it was not a nudist beach!)
Back home and back at work now. Thanks so much for all the comments on my last post about the beach and body confidence.
I first looked at those pictures of me in my costume and thought urgh, overweight. But I put myself out there and not one of you have said anything judgy - the only one who looks at them and thinks anything negative is me.
Being self-critical is a hard habit to change, so I looked again at the pictures today and tried to focus on something I liked about my shape. Very slowly my distorted view changed and I saw the overall image rather than just narrowing in on the wobbly bits.
The same is true of you and your body. We need to look at the things we actually like about ourselves first and focus on those instead of going straight to the flabby bits and hating ourselves.
How many family pictures have you deleted or cropped yourself out of because you thought you looked awful?
I am so guilty of this.

And, how many times have you sat there and said you were too tired, or 'just fine watching' instead of jumping up and playing with the kids?
The kids will play and have fun anyway, but that memory will never include mum running round the park playing chase or jumping in the pool on holiday and laughing with them.
Because you were just fine watching.

God forbid anybody should look at you and think something unflattering about your shape were you ever to get up and enjoy life. So, you sit it out.
There are so many memories and photographs of me that could have been but never will be, because I thought I looked awful.
But that stops right now.
The menopause has given me a lot of things I would prefer not to have; insomnia, bloating, pissing, farting, weight gain, anxiety, itchy skin, facial hair. It really is a shit shower! But this strange confidence, this 'feck it and feck you' attitude is an added, unexpected bonus that has given me the chance to get myself in those family photographs and get making those memories that include me being right in the thick of things.

In case you were wondering, the lady on the beach in front of me, did not get up off her chair and her small children eventually stopped calling for her to join them in the sea, and had lots of fun and giggles with their dad.
She never moved, but she watched them all the time.
When they are older and remember that day by the sea, they will remember dad playing with them and it will be as if their mum was never there.
Yet I bet she organised that holiday, washed everything, packed everything and wanted to join in so much it hurt.
This summer, be the lady in the surf with a smile on her face.
You deserve it. You are worth it.

Favourite comment:
Karen: I have just stuck my costumes back in the cupboard and got the bikini's out after reading this, you are so right…most of the time the only people who bother what we look like is ourselves. Thank you for giving me the incentive.

Sarah 1 Posh 0

2nd July 2023

Just back home having been hoofed out for the weekend by our eldest daughter, who wanted a party to celebrate turning 22 without her mother going round putting down coasters, rearranging the scatter cushions and screeching 'hands off my fucking gin!'

We have come back to a cul-de-sac of cross looking neighbours, a dishwasher full of glasses, and a house much cleaner than the one we left behind, so it must have been a good night.

We stayed in a charming dog friendly cottage.

I always read the visitor book and the comments were hilarious:

'There was no freezer so my six mince and onion microwave meals defrosted'

'The ironing board cover didn't fit properly'

'The lawn was dry'

'The birds were noisy'

I felt like writing 'fuck off and get a life' under all of these.

We stopped off at the local shop and purchased our supplies. Husband had been for a run and was chafing in a delicate area. He asked me to buy Sudocreme.

I chucked vodka, coke and Tia Maria into the basket. I had been bitten so in went some extra strong Piriton - the proper knock out stuff. I looked for something to ease the chafing for husband and grabbed some Vaseline.

The chap at the counter raised his eyebrows at my shopping and glanced to make sure I had been caught on CCTV while surreptitiously making a note of our number plate. Masses of booze, sleep inducing drugs and Vaseline! All I needed was a spade and some gaffer tape.

We briefly parked next to some playboys and their blondes (with obligatory 6ft legs) leaning on their Ferrari's and Lamborghini's so that my husband, (driving my Mokka) could reinsert his hearing aid and listen to me moan about my varicose vein.
I do not need a hearing aid and so I clearly heard him say 'my life is shit' as he floored the Mokka to a sedate 45 miles an hour.

I was feeling very un-menopausal so ignored his salty comment.

After a fabulous couple of days, which were not courtesy of the Vaseline, thank you very much - my trap door is exit only - we had a final lovely lunch in a dog friendly pub.

We had booked and checked that it was OK to have dogs inside.
Our dogs were knackered and flopped down, out of sight under our table.

Some very loud, very posh people sat down nearby. It took them three minutes to get a sentence out because their vowels were so extended. They were so loud that we all had to endure their conversation whether we wanted to or not. We finished our dinner; husband stood and took the dogs out to the car. The very posh woman had her back to me, saw our dogs going outside and said, very loudly:
'I do like dogs but I wish people would eat with them outside'
So, I said, equally loudly:
'I do like posh people but I wish they would eat outside'
Then I stuck my nose in the air and flounced off.
Sarah 1 Posh 0

The menopause vs trains.
10th July 2023
On our recent trip to London, my daughter and I had to stand on the train for almost the entire journey down from Shropshire. It was a hot day and our armpits knew it. We were sweating like a nun in a sex shop.
I started people watching and found myself being surprisingly generous.
The guy talking oh so loudly on his phone kept wiping his sweaty hands dangerously close to the crotch area of his pants. His voice went up a few octaves at one point as the train jolted vigorously and his paw slipped unexpectedly. But he had a wedding ring on so somebody loved him.
Lap top man was bashing away on the keyboard groaning, sighing, huffing, shoving the laptop away in exasperation and looking up occasionally with a hang dog expression, as if expecting sympathy from those of us forced to stand. I tried to smile encouragingly but he frowned and crouched over his laptop once more.
The train jolted on. Couples sat ignoring each other in favour of their phones, occasionally nudging each other to take a forced smiley selfie, then bent their heads once more, a twenty something jammed out to music only she could hear, a bloke with quite a large belly kept hoisting his T shirt up to treat us to the sight of him scratching his rather large hairy belly and then inspecting his fingernails.
His partner sat next to him eating crisps whilst somehow never closing her mouth.
Every now and then the internal sliding door would woosh open and we would all be treated to a blast of pungent stale toilet odour.
But none of this mattered, I was in a zen mood, happy and calm and at peace with the world, trying to find the best in everybody.

This smiley, happy and somewhat bewildering mood lasted for a whole five minutes before the real me kicked in and I stopped playing nice.

I looked at loud phone man and dreamt of showing the device up his arse, but sadly, he was using his arse to talk out of so it was otherwise engaged.

I wished I could ask him not to keep trying to feel his lad in public. If he must root around that much for it, then it is not worth finding.

Lap top man. No one gives a flying shit. Stop huffing and puffing and looking up at us as if your piles are hurting. You have got a seat on a busy train so shag off with yourself. Out of spite I leant down a few times and made sure he got a nice whiff of armpit.

Couples! Try putting your phones down and talking to each other instead of telling everyone on social media how much fun you are having, when the opposite is clearly true. You look as miserable as sin.

Dancing girl – keep dancing darling, never lose that spirit.

T shirt man, just fucking stop it, I do not want to look at your huge hairy belly. I have got one of my own to scratch and sniff, if I so choose, thank you very much. And please, tell your wife to close her great giant gob when she is eating. Looking at a mouthful of fillings, yellow teeth and mushed up pickled onion monster munch whilst being forced to inhale the smell of train bog is a new low, and one I never wanted to reach.

And, finally, train companies – put some more carriages on for the love of God. We are fucking customers not cattle.

It is not a crime

11th July 2023

Instead of looking in the mirror and hoping to see myself as I was at 25 years old only to be crushed by the reality, I am going to try to look in the mirror and expect to see a soon-to-be-52-year-old, knee deep in middle age shit.

And I am going to be a bit kinder to her.

All she did was get a bit older.

It is not a crime to put on weight.

It is not a crime to have a roll of flab.

It is not a crime to have a saggy bum, dimply thighs, bingo wings, a moustache and flaps that flop out of your swimsuit.

It is not a crime to fart the national anthem.

It is not a crime to lose control of your pelvic floor or have a dried-up fanny.

It is not a crime to age.

And it is not a crime to look different to how you did 30 years ago.

It is fucking normal!

I am tired of seeing celebrities in the media who are getting older without actually aging.

It is not real. It gives unrealistic expectations and it can make us normal women and men feel shitty and even ashamed that we have not held it together and kept the bodies and faces we had 25 years ago.

But feck all that!

We are fabulous and 100% real.

We are all gorgeous.

Give your achy hip a rub, pluck your nose and your chin and be proud of yourself.

Be kind to yourself, you just got a bit older, that is all.

Favourite comment from Suzanne:

In Australia you are a star if you can burp or fart any tune.

Summer Loving

14th July 2023

Summer when you were younger…out with your friends hitting the bars and clubs having the time of your life in tiny skirts and pretty crop tops.
You looked a million dollars.

The end of the night draws near, you know this because everyone forms a circle and starts kicking the shit out of each other under the guise of dancing to Come on Eileen, or, if you were at a wedding, New York New York.
You stagger out, have a dirty donner or a spud u like, take your shoes off and head home.

Over time, your miniskirts move further back into your wardrobe until, some years down the line, you realise with a pang of nostalgia and sadness that they no longer fit. To be frank; they will not get over the thigh of one leg, and so, like many other beloved items of clothing, the cute little flirty skirts go to the charity shop.
No point keeping them for 'one day' you might be deluded but you are not deranged.
Because you now live in jeans, several sizes bigger than you swore you would become.
Getting your legs out is reserved for 30-degree heat when you are left with no option other than to wear shorts or smell your own crotch burning.

To prepare the legs you have an argument with a razor, unblock the drains, apply some fake tan over your varicose veins - because making them orange and streaky renders the blue snakes invisible - and then paint your toenails because you cannot be arsed to remove the half grown out polish still there from 3 months ago.

The shorts cannot be too short in case a hairy flap or a piss
pad pops out to say hi.

Wearing a crop top is the stuff of fantasy, the closest you
have come to a crop top was wearing a nursing bra 21 years
ago, so you throw on a baggy t shirt and spend the day
wafting it in and out in front of you. Like a fan.
You would love not to wear a bra and let the girls free fall,
but the under boobs sweat slick is visible from space, so a
bra it is.
Armpits, boobs and groin are sprayed with anti-perspirant,
the process repeated every five minutes. It makes you sneeze
so you cross your legs and realise you have chafed.
Vaseline is applied to the top of your thighs to stop the chub
rub and you spritz perfume round your crotch to disguise the
highly sexual aroma of petroleum jelly and sneezed on piss
pad.

Yes, you are now a middle-aged lady.
And, with a smile on your face and a twinkle in your good
eye, you still look a million dollars

Darkness

25th July 2023

Author's note: Very recently, and for a number of reasons, I have found myself in a very dark place, made of lead, full of despair and unable to cope with any other emotion except nothingness.

Part of this, as I have since discovered when writing this book, is that my Mirena coil stopped releasing hormones into my system in around mid-June.

This caused a hormonal crash in mid-July.

Another reason, I believe, is that I had recently visited the area where I spent my childhood and come face to face with the past.

In this chapter I talk about abuse I suffered as a young girl. Although not the sole reason for this most recent slide into darkness, one can never underestimate the strength it takes to wear someone else's filth on you every day. This diary entry starts with me recounting our recent visit back home:

I have previously referred to my childhood abuse experience, at the hands of my primary school headmaster in the changing rooms of the swimming pool.

I have talked about my visit to the hairdresser, where I asked the hairdresser to 'make me look like a boy.' My eight-year-old self mistakenly believing that my abuser would not want me any more if he thought I was a boy.

The hairdresser's is now somebody's home, but when we drove past, I swear I saw myself as a young child sitting there having my hair cut off. In my eyes it was still a hairdresser's and I had to blink several times to shake the image.

After he retired from school, he got a job in the payment booth at the local wildlife park. The payment booth at the wildlife park was the last place I saw him; there he was leering down at me when we went on a trip a year or two after he had retired.

My husband and I went to the wildlife park on this recent visit, and the wooden payment booths were still there, unchanged after all this time. I was fixated on them, almost transfixed. I could not take my eyes off them, but I made by husband manoeuvre the car to one of the more modern booths.
Since then, flashbacks and nightmares have crept in, vivid and detailed, weighing me down like a hand on my shoulder that I cannot shake. Although the hairdresser's and the payment booth were the trigger, the flashbacks are always in the changing room.
This is why I believe that women should have a safe space to get undressed, be it the swimming pool, the clothes store, the spa or the gym.
The sight of male genitals in a place where you are only expecting to see other women is too triggering for an awful lot of females, especially if you are undressed and vulnerable. If you have transitioned into a woman and have had your male parts removed, then come on in.
But I do not want to see an adult male's penis and bollocks in the ladies changing room. Equal rights for everybody should not mean women's rights are trampled on and our very genuine fears pushed aside under the banner of inclusivity.

I am not saying all men are rapists or sexual offenders – far from it. But all women have been, at best scared shitless, at worse a victim of a sexual crime.
I know a lot of people, especially the younger generation, will disagree with me and that is OK, I accept have a lot to learn. I expect to get shouted down and that is OK too. The

loudest voices do not always speak for the majority. I did not have a voice as an eight-year-old, but I think I deserve to be heard now, and I think my opinion as a sexual abuse survivor should be considered when we debate about the use of female changing rooms.

Please seek help if you are suffering, it is available, and, trust me, it does help.
It was not your fault; it is not your shame to carry around and, at the very fecking least, you deserve to have a safe space to change when you go shopping.

Sisterhood
Thursday July 27th 2023

Today my little sister turns 50. She is beautiful and dazzling.
But just writing that she is 50 makes me realise how much
older I am than I feel.
I get annoyed that my knee aches and my hip hurts. I get
frustrated that my tummy gets in the way when I bend down
to shave my big toes. I stretch in the morning and everything
creaks and cracks.
I remember birthdays when my sister and I were younger,
wearing our 1970's NHS pink glasses and pudding bowl
haircuts, the lovely big cake, the parties and the friends.
Happy, carefree days before mobile phones, iPads, social
media.
We went out on our bikes and came back when we were
hungry. We taped the top 40 on a Sunday, we played with
Sindy and Girls World. If we hurt ourselves, we had a Dettol
or TCP bath and a cup of Lucozade.
We took the glass pop bottles back to the corner shop and
10 pence would buy you a whole bag of sweets.
A Curly Wurly was a foot long, black jacks and fruit salads
were half a pence and we bought Judy and Bunty comics for
ourselves, and the Beano for our Dad.
You could buy Spangles and Pacers and flavoured Toffo's.
We were always out at somebody's house and the neighbours
all knew and looked out for each other. I looked out for my
little sister because that is what we did, even if we sometimes
did not want to.
You morph into teenagers and make your own friends, you
grow up and go your own way, as you should.
But that sisterly bond, formed through childhood runs deep.
I look at my own girls now, getting ready to go out together,
laughing and giggling, so young and so beautiful and I hope

time slows a little bit for them while they are in this wonderful phase of their lives, free from the burdens and responsibility that age brings.

And then I look at an old couple trying to use the cashpoint machine opposite my office. Hunched over and supported by walking sticks, baffled by the ever-changing technology. All they want is to go into a warm branch of the bank and have a chat with a nice cashier and take some money out. But the branch has closed. So now, they balance awkwardly in the rain, trying to keep the walking stick propped up with an elbow whilst they root around for a cash card, peering at the screen and entering their pin with shaking hands before they shuffle slowly and carefully away.

It is a reminder that life moves quickly. In the blink of an eye, my sister has gone from turning 5 to turning 50. Despite the creaking and the aching, we middle aged folk really are in the prime of our lives, and I am going to try harder to remember that.

Cantankerous Cleaning
Thursday 3rd August 2023

There are varying levels of anger that you experience in your life:
Baby anger – wailing because you want food or your bum wiping.

Toddler anger – pushing those boundaries by having a full-on meltdown in Tesco, uncaring that you are making a holy scene, and making your body go ridged and immovable in a way that you will never be able to do again, until you die.

Teenage anger – shouting, hating everybody, door slamming, music blaring hormonal angst, that nobody understands and nobody over the age of 25 has ever experienced.

Married anger – I love you but get the fuck out of my face.

Mum anger – I will give you something to cry about, Harry Styles my arse, I do not care what everyone else's mum says, the PTA can shag off with their fecking cake sale, in my house Kylie will eat fish fingers and fecking well like them, because I said so, slam that door again and I will pack your bags lady etc.

But nothing, NOTHING comes close to menopausal anger.
It is like you have been reincarnated as a wasp.
The difference is that you actually like being angry.
Everything pisses you off and you basically hate everybody, so why not channel that anger, and make it work for you?
You drive angry, you shop angry and you cook angry. I think I even go to the toilet angry.
But there is a positive: angry cleaning.

I hoover angry – it is great – I am so enraged that the venom
spills out of me and down the hoover which responds with
vigorous glee and snaffles every last dog hair, crumb and
speck of dust, leaving the floor spotless.
Ditto cleaning the bathroom, nasty, angry scrubbing is good
for the soul and leaves the shower gleaming.
I clench my teeth, arm myself with the toilet brush and take
out my fury on the skid marks. It is therapeutic. Especially as
the chances are they were my skids, the result, no doubt, of a
giant meno shit.
And when it is done, I have a G & T and wait for someone
to leave a dirty plate out and piss me off all over again.
I swear, angry housework is the way forward; I am thinking
of starting a cleaning business and calling it menopausal
maids – the fuming fumigators.

Even my ego is hairy.
Monday 7th August 2023

I was reading through the reviews of my book, stroking my
ego – even that is hairy - when I was suddenly struck by just
how many ladies say they felt alone before I came along with
my big mouth and dry fandango bleating about the
menopause.

I did not know what to expect when I first started getting
symptoms. Friends of mine had experienced hot flushes, but
they seemed to cope OK with everything.
So, when I had a few hot flushes at the age of 48, I flapped
my arms, mopped my brow, and thought 'bring it on! I am
so ready to not have periods and all that crampy, bloating
every month.'
I was an innocent.
A menopause virgin whose friends had only been to first
base.
Me? I went all the way with fucking bells on.
I like to think I took one for the team and had all their
symptoms, all at once.
My fanny went dry. Apologies for blurting that out, but there
is no pleasant way to make that announcement! It just
happened. I would still want sex and feel sexy, but the
message did not reach below my waist. It was like I had dried
up inside out.
I put weight on, literally two stone piled on from nowhere,
and I was not exactly a stick insect before my hormones
went haywire. I felt like a blob of lard.
Eventually I stopped feeling sexy, because rummaging
around for a tube of lube and being able to feel myself
wobbling, whilst doing the deed, well, it was not exactly a
turn on.

I felt anxious, depressed, tearful, angry, confused, and sad. I just felt very sad and sorry for myself that I was experiencing all this horror and nobody else really got it.

I wanted to wear bright red and have RAGE scrawled across my forehead so that people would notice me and say' oh bless, she is having a hard time with the menopause, let's not fuck with that.' And keep out of my way.

Or give me a G & T and some tissues.

But, because we got too good at keeping things in and coping, nobody really spoke about what happens when the menopause drains the life out of you and how it feels to fall apart.

And that is how I see the menopause. You fall apart. Bits of you fall away, your memory fucks off only to return in fragments at 3am when you suddenly remember that name you were trying to think of. Your pelvic floor packs up and leaves town, leaving a floppy, flappy trap door in its place that can just about hold in a sneeze, but two sneezes, and, God forbid, a cough, is out of the question.

Your self-worth and sense of confidence vanishes: You are not who you thought you were because, unlike everybody else, you are not coping well with the menopause, you feel lost, old, scared, and angry. And pissy.

Well, I am here to tell you that what you feel is perfectly normal. There is no right or wrong way to have your menopause, or peri-menopause. You do not have to have the body of a 12-year-old or an Olympic athlete and a smile on your face.

You can, and probably will, have at least one roll of flab - you will get quite fond of it eventually, giving it gentle slaps of encouragement.

Your hormones are fleeing your body – it is like being a teenager in reverse, and your ovaries are literally shrivelling

up and dying – so it is no wonder we feel bewildered and
bemused.
If men saw their balls shrivel up and drop off, I think we
would be quite sweet and understanding about it – and,
guess what? – most men will be sympathetic to you if you
explain what is happening to you. They are not mind readers
and we women are far too good at clamming up and being
'fine' when, really, we are anything but.
It is a difficult time, you are hot, crabby, itchy, you have an
unwanted moustache and chin stubble. You feel as sexy as a
dose of the clap and even your big toes are hairy. Your legs
look like enormous grey hams.
In short, you have fallen out of love with yourself.
And that is a shame.
Because you are still you, and you deserve to be loved.
Knowing you are not alone is a fabulous feeling, you can
start to feel better about yourself and even learn to laugh at
all this shit being thrown at you.
So, if you are just starting out on this journey, I hope you
find your people and that you can talk and laugh and forgive
yourself for changing.
And if, like me, you have been on this roller coaster for a
couple of years, I hope that you have reached that stage
where you do not give much of a shit what people think of
you, because that is hugely empowering.
And the sex life? That gets better too. Once I told my
husband how I was feeling he understood that I was not
rejecting him, I was embarrassed of myself.
He has been very understanding and I see that he loves me
and it does not matter what shape or size I am.
Turns out I do not have much of a filter, and am very good
at blurting out how I feel, so we laugh a lot and that brings
us closer together. He thinks I am sexy and that makes me
feel confident.

And if he had not responded like that, I think I would have packed my bags and gone to Greece.
Because we women are awesome and we deserve the best. So, stand up with a very loud fart, and go face the world, knowing you are, after all, just wonderfully normal.

Great auntie goat chin

Tuesday 8th August 2023

Back in the day the only depiction of a menopausal woman on TV was Les Dawson's Cissy and Ada: wonderful jowly faced, plain, heaving bosom larger ladies who could barely whisper the word 'change.' The bar was pretty low, so it was not difficult to feel glamorous and attractive in comparison.

How many of us had a great auntie goat chin, a relative we were a bit wary of kissing, who had a fondness for sherry, clearly was not bothered about her whiskers and smelt of wee?

But now, we have any number of stunning women with incredible faces and bodies talking about the menopause or just being out there, winning at everything, the same age or older than me, looking fabulous.

If I start to feel down, I remind myself that their menopause is not the same as my menopause. In my world a six pack lives in the pantry and is full of crisps. I like to get in from work and flop on the sofa. I might get up to make dinner, I might say I cannot be arsed and order a take away. I might get the hoover out or I might kick the dog hair under the sofa and save it for another day.

I am a million women feeling old, knackered, fat and generally a bit fecked off with a dry fanny and an arse that I no longer pretend to have control over. It farts when it wants to no matter the consequence for its poor owner. I am a million women who struggle at work trying to remember what they are supposed to be doing and so spend the day trying to pluck that bastard stubborn chin hair out instead.

I am a million women struggling to sleep at night on a sea of sweat and a million women suffering with rage, anxiety, and depression. I am a million women who are just a little bit normal, and thank goodness for us.

I am a million women who look in the mirror and wonder who the feck that old bag is staring back at me with a slack jaw and a look of surprise on her face? It cannot possibly be you because you are still 25 and have glowing dewy skin, yet this person is a blotchy, sweaty lady. You slather on face cream, foundation, blusher, highlighter, eye liner, mascara, draw your eyebrows back on.
Success!
Along comes a hot flush and sweats it all off again.
You pluck your nostril and sneeze.
You have remembered to wear a piss pad in your giant grey pants, but it was quite a vigorous sneeze.
You sniff as close to your crotch as your roll of flab will allow.
This is not a position the younger you ever anticipated being in – vaguely sniffing in the direction of your own crotch to see if your pad will last a bit longer or not.
It dawns on you that you could be great auntie goat chin without the sherry.
Luckily you do not like sherry so you will never be the same as her.
No, you are great auntie goat chin with a G & T.
And you are awesome.

Dumbledore's Beard.
Wednesday 9th August 2023

Further to yesterday's post when I wrote about bending over to try and sniff my crotch area to see if the piss pad could survive a little bit longer, I got to thinking of all the other things I do now that I never dreamt would be coming down the line at me.

Back when I was pre-menopausal and still had a reasonably slim, firm body I never once imagined I would have to heft a shelf of flab out of the way in order to see if my growler needed pruning.

And back when I did have a nice, firm body I also had a tidy, trim bush. Not too little that I looked pre-pubescent and not too much that it could be used a dental floss. Did I ever imagine I would look at it and think 'fuck off, I'm not up to attacking that?' No. I kept it nice. Now it is either all off, save for a few grey wiry ones that defeat the scissors, or it is as full and wild as Dumbledore's beard.

And my feet were quite pretty with polished nails and a bit of a tan. Now I have six-month-old half grown out nail varnish, soles the same texture as sandpaper, a sun burn 'V' from flip flops, a big toe with a goatee and yeti hair on the top of my feet.

My legs were quite nice and shapely, not chunky grey hams with a varicose vein snaking up the calf, looking for all the world like a map of the motorway network.

I used to be quite patient and pleasant but now, well, everyone is a bell end specifically put on earth to piss me off.

I really do not know what has happened and I certainly was not expecting all this horror. But fuck it all 'til Friday; I am not twenty any more, Christ! I will never see fifty again, but I have enjoyed myself and I am still enjoying myself. I have laughed more than I have cried – even now with the bastard menopause – and we cannot come back and live our lives again so let us make the best of what we have got.

I know there are times when you feel so down it is hard to even get out of bed, you are disappointed that you have changed and despondent that you cannot be bothered to do anything much about it. But it is not our fault we were born women, and we need to stop being so hard on ourselves and expecting to be perfect. We are fine, just the way we are.

So let the 'fro below grow, eat the crisps, drink the gin and stop beating yourself up for not having a model body. If you see Amanda Holden, Davina or Liz Hurley in the paper looking fabulous in a bikini, scrunch it up and save it for kindling. Or use it to line the cat litter tray. Balls to them.

Marigolds
Monday 14th August 2023.

On Saturday a friend of mine was 50 – he is one of the
youngest of us - and he optimistically invited his aged mates
on a 12-hour, 12 pub crawl through the beautiful Ironbridge
Gorge, which is where most of us in attendance are lucky
enough to call home.
One pint per pub was the objective which went flying out of
the window the minute the sun came out and we decided to
be typically British and make the most of it by having 2 pints
in a beer garden by the river in-between the showers.
The more pints we drank the more shite we talked.
Gone are the days of sex, drugs and rock and roll.
No, our conversation inexplicably turned to wearing
marigolds, which got the birthday bot excited – I didn't like
to ask why, but he was keen to know how many pairs I had
and what uses I put them to - followed by the loading of the
dishwasher.
I personally do not see how difficult it is to obey the design
of the appliance and stack the plates in the fecking slots, the
cups on the tray above and the knives and forks in their
holder. But throw in a large bowl or a baking tray and it all
goes to shit in our house. Stuff is thrown and rammed in
every which way, with little or no hope of it actually coming
out clean.
Half the plates then come out with food sandblasted onto
them which means I have to invoke the Brillo Pad. This puts
me in mind of my aging growler, reminding me I have yet to
trim it, and makes scrubbing the plates all the more
unpleasant.
In keeping with the high drama of our lives, we then turned
our conversation to composting.

We were 4 pints in by this point, the birthday boy was keen to point out he had two bins and Mrs A remind us that we must fork our compost.

But at least we did not talk about crochet.

At pint 5 I gate-crashed a hen do and borrowed their willy deely boppers for a photo op with my friends. None of us can remember why.

Just to enforce my middle age credentials, I proudly showed my friends the pattern I had ordered for my new curtains.

At pub 6 I cast a blurry eye around for my husband. He had drunk a fair few pints to keep up with the 'lads' and had been complaining that he would be up peeing all night and might as well sleep on the toilet, which alarmed me because that is where I was intending to pitch myself for the night. After 6 pints of lager, I could pee like a race horse, had a farting competition with my friend in the next loo and even nodded off briefly.

The next morning, with a banging head I thought back to our night and everything that had taken place.

Marigolds

The scared art of loading the dishwasher

Composting

Willy deely boppers

Curtains

Farting

Nana napping mid wee

Just as I was despairing about being boring, middle aged housewife cliché I looked at my phone.

Before I had crashed into bed, I had sent a message to the birthday boy which said 'great night, I'll be round with my marigolds tomorrow' followed by the finger emoji and a winking face.

There is life in the old dog yet.

Are you with me?
Tuesday 15th August 2023

This month marks 25 years since David and I set first eyes
on each other; we got engaged after 9 weeks and next year is
our silver wedding anniversary – which fecks with my head
because I remember taking my basin haircut and best long
dress to silver wedding anniversary parties in the 1970's
which were full of old people.
I remember that first flush of love when you spend ages
getting ready and smell gorgeous. Every inch of you is
slathered in body lotion, de-fuzzed and you glow with desire.
Now I glow like sweaty lava as I boil over with hot flush, and
I ask my husband to smell my armpits in case I have gone
nose blind. I still sniff my own pants though.
When did this transition take place? When did I decide it was
OK to shove my pit in my husband's face and ask him if I
whiffed?
Maybe it was the same day that I picked my knickers up off
the floor and used them to dust the dresser in the bedroom
on the way to the wash basket?
Perhaps it was the same day that I accepted I would have to
wear a piss pad all day, or the day I discovered hair growing
on the top of my feet?
Was this the same day I bent over in public and let out a fart
of such tremendous force the entire room, including me,
thought I must have shit myself?
What about the day I decided I could no longer be arsed to
pluck my chin and borrowed David's razor to give it the
once over? There is no going back after that.
Or was it the day I realised my growler liked to ensnare bits
of toilet roll, twirl them up and spit them out again? It is
especially fond of doing this during sex.

Did all these things happen on the same day or was it so
gradual that I hardly noticed?
Little by little, my feminine dignity is being
stripped away. I am fighting the good fight but, holy fuck, it
is exhausting being a woman sometimes.
But while I am still able, I will keep spraying myself with
Febreze, blaming my husband or the dog for my farts,
excusing myself to the loo after two sneezes, putting my
make up on, washing all my hair, removing my loo roll cling
ons and rocking the sweaty yeti look.
Are you with me?

Sandblasting and sex
Thursday 17th August 2023
Tomorrow the husband and I are off for the weekend to a
lovely little log cabin with a private hot tub. It will be our
wedding anniversary on Sunday.

This means sex which means I must prepare.

I have let myself go and grow this summer. In my defence,
the weather has been so awful that the chances of showing
more than an ankle have been few and far between.

But my husband and I are not prude Victorians and I dare
say I will be flashing more than an ankle at him this weekend.
So, yesterday, I did the great shave of the legs – it has been a
fortnight since I did them last and I had man legs. Hat's off
to anyone who is OK with a hairy leg, but I looked like I was
wearing furry trousers and it was not attractive.
Legs were followed by armpits, feet and, alas, nipples.
I then exfoliated vigorously, trying to make the lardy bits
vanish.

Stepping out of the shower, looking like I had been
sandblasted, I tried to rub away the gritty bits of the
exfoliator with the towel but managed to deposit most of it
in my bum crack.
Finally, I lathered my body with moisturiser.

Tonight, I will tackle the great grey growler or the 'for below.
I have a bin bag and Mr Muscle on standby.
Tomorrow morning, I will shave everywhere again, pluck my
chin and wax off my moustache.

Then I will dig out my little nightie, make sure I have packed the lube and, finally, after two days of preparation, I will be ready for spontaneous sex.

My husband will give his lad a quick wash – ever hopeful – and that is him good to go.

We really do get the shitty end of the stick, don't we?

Favourite comment:

Sweary wee me: At least you were not STUPID enough to try home wax strips! I nearly stuck a flap to my elbow and lost a strip somewhere along the line…which made itself very apparent when I stood up from the bathroom floor, because I had fucking SAT ON IT and pretty much glued my hoop shut! Never again.

Burn baby burn

Saturday 19th August 2023

Here we are on our romantic forest retreat weekend away.

I booked for petals to be strewn on the bed.

I also booked for us both to have an in-cabin massage.

My husband shit himself on learning this because he has booked precisely feck all.

This means I have a guilt-ridden slave at my beck and call all weekend.

The petals looked lovely but ended up ensnared in my bum crack and hairy hoo hoo that I never did find the time to tackle.

We took the dogs on a massive walk first thing this morning to tire them out, so that we could be massaged in peace.

Safe to say, after two hours of following my nose, we were hopelessly lost in Delamere Forest. After blindly stumbling through bracken and massive pine trees that all look the fucking same, we were pathetically grateful to find ourselves somehow on the Peter Rabbit trail, which we assumed led back to civilisation.

I do not know if the Peter Rabbit trail is designed for Bear shagging Grylls or not but it was torturously long.

The thighs on the inside of my jeans had decided to split so I had bare thigh chafing bare thigh, a fire risk, frankly, in a forest, and we were now 15 minutes late for our lovely massage appointment.

Finally, we burst out of the forest, me walking like I had been astride a horse for a week, sweating from everywhere and looking like a boiled crab.

Husband looked for all the world like he had just sauntered up the road.

With apologies to the massage ladies, we stripped off and collapsed on the massage beds.

By now I was gasping and dripping and wanted a month-
long ice-cold shower, a tub of Sudocreme on my inner thighs
and a sleep.
But I had to be all relaxed and lovely for my massage.
My face stuck to the tissue used to line the hole in the table.
I saw my own sweat drip down onto the floor.
I put my arms above my head and smelt my own armpits.
I was desperate to fart.
I was as relaxed as a coiled spring.
My humiliation was complete when my therapist had to
BLOT my sweaty back with kitchen roll before she could
start.
For the love of Mary.
But it was lovely and afterwards, for no other reason than to
be spiteful, I used my husband's moisturiser to sooth my
burning chafage.
Welcome to 24 years of marriage. All that preparation to be
romantic, and I manage to chafe my inner thighs so much
that if husband even looks at me with a raised eyebrow my
hairy flaps will entwine together and shut up shop.

Wear the marquee
Monday 21ˢᵗ August 2023

Dear lovely lady,

You are reading this and feeling alone and confused. You
have changed and you do not particularly like your new body
or the fact that your brain is running at 50% capacity.
No matter what exercise you take or diets you follow you are
flabbier than you used to be. You feel unattractive and
unsure.
The menopause has crashed into your lovely life and made it
all a little bit shit.
Your husband's loud breathing has you eyeing up the knife
drawer.
The dishwasher being incorrectly loaded sends you into an
orbit of fury.
You feel martyred and permanently pissed off that nobody
notices how crap everything has become for you.
Just getting out of bed takes a huge effort.
You have bingo wings.
You are sweaty.
The only person who understands you is the dog.
You itch so much you feel like you have fleas.
You have grown an extra, unwanted chin and it is prone to a
crop of stubborn stubble.
You forget what you are saying and what you are doing.
Farts just blow out of you without warning or control.
There are so many different things happening to you that it is
hard to keep track, never mind hold down a job, stick a smile
on your face and keep everyone else together.
You feel like you are lost.
Everyone is a prick.
You say Fuck far more than you used to.

Sex is for people who feel attractive, confident, and worthy.
Guess what?
You are normal, normal, normal.
And you are attractive, confident, and worthy – you have just
been buried under the menopause.
You are going through the worse time in a woman's life and
you are being bombarded by images in the media telling us
that we should still be slim, sexy and glamorous and make
the effort.
Fuck that for Christmas.
Wash your hair, put your make up on and wear something
you feel good in.
Even if it is a marquee.
You are the girl we all want to go out for a drink and a giggle
with.
You are still you.
Be kind to yourself.

Love, Sarah x

Sorry
Wednesday 23rd August 2023

Today I am going to write about my husband, he has gone grey since we married, needs to wear glasses all the time now, and has recently been fitted with hearing aids. But he has kept fit and healthy, is still gorgeous and sexy. His mind and body remain alert and active, and his kind and patient temperament have been unchanged by time.
I guess I want to say sorry to him.
I am not the same girl he married.
She was a slim, glowing, happy young thing, bright eyes and optimistic. She wore shirt skirts, was flirty and playful. She kept herself fit and her mind was sharp.
Now, I cry when I cannot unwrap an opal fruit and have to wear his boxer shorts because my flabby thighs chafed so much, I gave myself a friction burn.
I mean, I am almost unrecognisable from the person he married!
My optimism has turned to anxiety and depression.
My happiness has turned to rage.
My bright eyes have droopy eyelids and a death glare.
My glowing skin is boiled and sweaty.
My slim figure has ballooned.
My short skirts are pyjamas with elasticated waists.
My sharp mind feels dull and foggy.
My fitness has plummeted and now I feel tired all the time.
In every possible way I have changed.
And I do not think I have given my husband enough credit for how difficult the menopause must be for him.
He walks about on eggshells and tries to help when he sees I am struggling.
He does not always say or do the right things, but he tries to understand and reassures me that he still loves me.

At times I have been convinced that he will leave, that he cannot possibly fancy me or find me attractive; however, that is all part of the anxiety and paranoia that hormonal changes can bring.

He has stuck around and he has done it with a smile on his face and his arm around me.

In the depth of these changes we are battling with, I am quite certain that we ladies do not always show our appreciation, but, for all the good guys out there – thank you for loving us when we could not love ourselves.

And if anyone out there has an ex- husband who did not stick around and buggered off with some young dolly bird, consider this: The menopause gets us all in the end, she will puff out, piss and fart just like the rest of us. And that bastard will get to live it all over again!

Wankhole
22nd August 2023

This is what you need to learn in school:
Girls, you will have periods for around 35 years which is shit.
You will have to pay for basic sanitary protection which is
grossly fucking unfair because it is a necessity and not a
luxury.
At some point, when you are bent double with period
cramps and have flooded your knickers yet again, you will
dream about the day your ovaries begin to shrivel and all this
blood and pain will fade.
You may even think that the menopause is a good thing.
This is Bullshit with bells on.
Parts of your body are now redundant – the reproductive
organs are literally dying inside of you and, as these organs
cease to function, your hormones send your body into a
tailspin of emotions.
Your default emotion will be rage.
You will feel angry for no other reason than you just want to
be angry.
You will feel like you are being boiled alive and sweat will
pour out of you from everywhere. Your ears will sweat, your
flaps will sweat. Your fucking knees will sweat.
Your head will go bright red. This will always happen in a
public place or when you give a serious, professional
presentation.
You will want to scream 'FUCK OFF' every five minutes.
None of your clothes will fit and you will feel flabby and
unattractive.
Your vagina will go dry.
You will forget what you are saying or doing while you are
shagging well saying it or doing it.
Your skin will feel dry and itchy.

Your sex drive will vanish, and is it any wonder when your fanny looks as attractive as an ancient dry turtle's head wearing a Brillo pad?

But, despite the leaking, creaking and sweating there is life in the old girl yet and this is my survival guide: You can fight back.

For the sake of your sanity, see the doctor and get HRT or anti-depressants to help with the low moods and anxiety. I am on anti-depressants, there is absolutely nothing to feel ashamed about or any stigma – my life would be awful if I did not have something to help calm and soothe my poor head.

Do not blame yourself - It is not our fault that our hormones have gone crazy.

Take herbal supplements – sage is really helping my hot sweats.

With the greatest of respect, tell the likes of Davina and Amanda Holden to fuck right off – they are clearly having a different menopause to the rest of us.

Try to love your new curves, shop for who you are not who you used to be.

Setting spray for make up is a God send and stops it all sliding off during a hot flush.

Go to the hairdressers and treat yourself to a cut and colour, ask them what will suit you.

Ask at the make up counter for advice on what will suit your face now that you are a bit older. I have been using fucking Heather Shimmer lipstick for 30 years and it looks awful on me now. I look like a corpse. Do not be afraid to change.

Buy lubricant in any flavour you fancy, and get yourself a Moregasm from Ann Summers or similar from Love Honey and some nice sexy nighties that cover the wobbly bits. You can get your sex drive back – the Moregasm will help. Oh boy, it helps!

Say 'FUCK OFF' every five minutes, it is good for your soul.
Menopause Tourette's will appear in all its glory whilst you
are driving – let it out loud and proud, you will not give a
shit and you will feel better for it.

WANKHOLE is one of my new favourites, it took me by
surprise but I like it.

Talk to your partner, talk to your friends, find a support
group, follow this page or others like it. You are not alone
and you never will be.

If you leak, like I do, wear a pad every day.

Don't stretch, jump, run or cough too much – Lord knows
which hole will erupt.

Laugh, cry, rant, smile, scream.

Do what you feel comfortable with. You are still you under
all these layers of shit.

But, please do not be tempted to peek a look at the Brillo
pad wearing ancient dry turtle! That really is depressing.

Baptism of fire
29th August 2023
This weekend we have been down south visiting my uncle. It is never easy because he has dementia and several other health conditions. None of it is his fault, of course, but he is no longer the lovely uncle I grew up with and so we all try to do our best and make sure he is safe and cared for.
It is a challenge; he is a stubborn, proud man, widowed and childless and very much in denial about the severity of his conditions. Anybody who has experience of a relative with dementia will know what I mean when I say it is exhausting, exasperating, and depressing.
You spend hours and hours going round in circles trying to persuade the patient that they need more help than they are willing to accept.
Loving a person with dementia is very difficult and frustrating, but you just keep trying, don't you?
Afterwards we met up with friends and spent many happy hours unwinding courtesy of several double gin and tonics. I won't lie; I felt the need to just be young, fit and free having been cramped up in my uncle's extremely unhealthy home.
So, we got very pissed.
We then slurred and staggered back to our B & B which turned out to be under the flightpath of Heathrow.
What followed was a night of torture: My wine addled husband needed a wee approximately every 20 minutes. Despite turning the light on he still managed to collide with every item of furniture in the room. At one point he fell in the shower.
If he wasn't up and about having a wee, he was up hunting for his heartburn medication, having a pill for his headache or snoring.

When I finally closed my eyes, the 747's starting taking off right above me.

Husband had been up and down all night and managed to wrench his shoulder. I had been tossing and turning all night and managed to wrench my neck.

By dawn we were groaning and creaking like a couple of nonagrians and made my uncle look positively glowing with health in comparison.

Back at home we were told that our daughter's boyfriend is completing a sports massage therapist course and needed volunteers to work on. I normally avoid anything with the word sport in it, but my neck was really painful so I put myself forward as a subject.

Oscar was under strict instructions not to inflict any sort of pain on me and was subjected to the vision of me in my yellow bra.

Immediately I started slapping him and squealing that he was being too hard. Massage oil was needed. Husband was dispatched to the bedside drawer and came down with oil called Love me hard, or thrust or something equally inappropriate.

My daughter's eye roll was as audible as Oscar choking back his vomit.

But as it was either that or Crisp n Dry, we opted for the sexy massage oil.

Ever the professional, Oscar got to work valiantly ignoring the fluid stream of curses I was unleashing in his direction. Husband looked on jealously as the 20-year-old male hands got to work on me, but only because he wanted a massage himself.

Poor Oscar then had to use thrust/love me hard oil on my husband's hairy arm and up to his shoulder to an accompaniment of groans and grunts that I thought sounded worryingly familiar.

Talk about a baptism of fire, I think we have successfully managed to put him off his chosen career for life.

Heatwave

Monday 4th September 2023

Ah, the early autumn heatwave. Mother nature at her finest
We have had a summer of shite weather which means we
have all stayed in and eaten crisps and chocolate and our
body hair has gone feral, safe in the knowledge that we need
not expose ourselves in the rain.

Just when we middle aged lasses think we can shove our
hoof chomping shorts and tee shirts that are as flattering to
rolls of flab as wearing clingfilm, to the back of the wardrobe
for another 9 months, along comes the sun and hot weather.
Instead of glorying in the elasticated leggings, extra wide calf
boots and tunic tops of autumn, I am now faced with my
summer wear once more.

Alas, I am bigger than I was as the start of the summer. This
means I have flap saddle bags hanging down from my shorts,
like squashed bollocks, and a rollover bulging over the
waistband.

But the heatwave also means vodka and lemonade in the
garden after work and sandwiches for tea because nobody
can be bothered to get up off their arses and cook.

It means my arms look like boiled pink hams and my toes
finally get shaved.

Everyone who has been on holiday abroad these last two
weeks gets to come back and smugly show off their lovely
glowing bodies instead of shivering and turning the central
heating on.

Boots will have to dig out all their Dove summer glow
instead of stocking the 3 for 2 Christmas shite and I will have
to sniff my arm pits every hour, just to check my new eco-
friendly roll-on is up to the job.

Mr Muscle drain unblocker will do a roaring trade as millions of hairy legs are shaved for the first time since June, and, in the UK, we Brits will all have the same conversation in every shop we go in:

'Lovely weather'

'It's about time'

'Shame about the kids going back'

'Enjoy it while it lasts'

Despite the heat, I will have to keep wearing my pyjama bottoms in bed because September is the month of the very big hairy spiders coming in the house and I don't want one eyeing up my hairy hoo hoo and thinking 'Mummy!' thank you very much.

I will get bitten and stung by every living flying insect on the planet as they enjoy one last feast of flesh before dying, and my legs will itch and swell up in a most attractive fashion. I will radiate a musky aroma of anti-histamine cream, intertwined with the scent of sweaty armpits whose deodorant is not quite working, plus whatever squashed bollock-like newly shaved saddle bags smell like.

None the less I am going to enjoy the sunshine, while it lasts.

Daddy Long Legs
6th September 2023

I just googled 'Daddy Long Legs' and this came up:

What is a daddy long legs? Usually, this is the colloquial
name given to a crane fly, those flies that are long of body
and much longer of leg, with bendy knees. Their name
reflects an affection towards the lanky insects.

Can I just state here and now that I have no affection
whatsoever for these bloody things. We have been plagued
by them in our house which means I had to sleep with the
windows shut last night to stop the spindly feckers coming
in.

Flying spiders! Whoever thought that would be a good idea?
At least it ups my husband's macho cred a notch because I
have to pathetically whimper to him to come and remove the
horrible, dancing, giant, flapping monsters.

Upstairs he came flexing his muscles and feeling manly, to
aid his damsel in distress, then, with both hands cupped
around the beast (the Crane Fly - the other beast was firmly
zipped away from anything that might bite it) he tripped over
my outstretched ankles and landed on top of me. With the
flying spider still in his hands.

I moved as if my bones had melted and slid out from under
him quicker than you can scream 'Get that fucker away from
me' which is, coincidentally, exactly what I did say. Except I
screamed it with a closed mouth in case the beast (either
one) saw my wide open mouth and took advantage.

As fast as we could tip them out of the window, more came in. Window closed. It was like sleeping in an oven. Who doesn't love that as a menopausal woman prone to night sweats? I put the fan on and pointed it directly at the bit that needed it the most.

After two minutes the fan just blew hot hair around. It was like have my pubes blow dried in a sauna.

Why, in this country, can't we have one week of lovely weather without some fecking plague of beasts descending?

I swear the wasps and mozzies have been flying around all summer bored shitless and starving. I get my legs out for 20 minutes in September and they are like 'Yay! Dinner time! Nom fucking Nom.' Roll on Autumn!

Moth balls
7th September 2023

Yesterday I wrote about Daddy Long Legs, and I wasn't
referring to the ridey dad at the school gate that you used to
eye up.
Lots of you made a comment about moths. I do not like
moths, never have. Butterflies yes. Moths no. Hairy,
powdery, creepy, fluttering feckers.
Here is my moth story…

Years ago, I lived in southwest France, a beautiful, rural place
surrounded by sunflowers and vineyards.

One hot, sultry night I was awoken from my slumber
because I needed a wee. Off I plodded. The bathroom
window was open. Halfway through my wee a heard what
could only be a helicopter hovering outside. The noise was
tremendous. The helicopter then came in and landed ON
MY HEAD.

The helicopter was a giant fucking moth.
I could not scream because I only had knickers on and my
mum and dad were sleeping nearby, as were my tiny children.
I did not want my dad to see me in just my knickers and I
didn't want to frighten my babies.

The huge moth fluttered and scratched around in my hair.
My wee turned into a frightened fart which turned into a shit.
The moth remained purring on my head which made me
panic.
The more I panicked the more my bowels turned to liquid
and emptied. I cramped and groaned while trying not to

move my head. It felt like a stream of lava erupting from me that would never end.

I fancied I would just melt into a pool of shit and sweat and be discovered in the morning as a pair of knickers with a giant moth looking smugly on.

Finally, in danger of apoplexy, I reached for the loo roll and did the necessary.
Just as I finished wiping, the loo roll came to an end.

With an instinct that I think only other women can understand, I changed the toilet roll with a giant moth on my head, no more capable of leaving a cardboard tube there for the next person than I was of flying to the moon.
I left the toilet.
The moth took fright and flew off my head.
I shut it in the loo and raced to wake my husband.
I hyperventilated the words 'Giant moth, head, shit, but loo roll got changed' and left my man to deal with it.

He actually rolled his eyes as if I was some half-wit prone to exaggerating.
The nerve of him. I've told him a million times that I never exaggerate.

He confidently opened the toilet door, looking like some cool, unflustered naked hero, fully expecting to see a tiny speck of a moth he could flick away.

Instantly he screamed, fled the bathroom, and ran away windmilling his arms with the moth in hot pursuit, bollocks and lad flapping everywhere.

I ran around, boobs flopping, not really knowing where I
was going but dancing like I was on hot bricks.

My Dad appeared in his boxers. We tried not to look at each
other.

He swatted the moth and stunned it so that we could release
it outside.
The moth was a death's head moth, the stuff of horror films.
I need the loo again just thinking about it, and, after seeing
my naked husband being chased by a giant Lepidoptera,
moth balls have a whole new meaning for me.

The last post (sort of).

10th September 2023

This is one of the last posts I will write before sending my diary entries off to the publisher and it feels fitting to talk about what a tough year it has been. Overall, this diary is a fun and light-hearted take on the menopause, but I know that many of us struggle so very much with all the symptoms.

In July I suffered from a very sudden and deeply disturbing bout of depression. It was a breakdown of my mind and body, and, in the space of a few hours, I found myself sobbing helplessly, quite unable to stop. It is no exaggeration to say I wanted to die.

My husband and I were at a festival and had to pack our stuff up and walk to meet my daughter; actually, my husband and friends packed our stuff up. I simply stood there crying with my friends trying to comfort me. In order to get to our daughter, we had to cross over the River Severn at Shrewsbury. I had to carry two fold-up chairs, with the straps over each shoulder, as my poor husband was already leaden with picnic hampers and bags.

As we crossed the bridge it occurred to me in the clearest possible way, that if I crisscrossed the chair straps across my body, they would not fall off me when I jumped in the river and their extra weight would help me sink quickly to the bottom.

I have never felt such despair, or such a certainty that leaving this world was the right thing to do. Perhaps it was the mothering instinct that stopped me, the thought of my daughter waiting in her car for a mother who would never come. But I didn't jump. Instead, I crossed the bridge, never taking my crying eyes off the river, and I wished I was in there, with the weeds and the water.

It is very hard to talk about depression, because when you are in the depths of despair, it feels comfortable and safe. The outside world is loud, and cheerful and bright, and your mind simply cannot cope with it all. So, you retreat. And you are sad that you have withdrawn, but you truly believe that everyone is better off just carrying on without you.

I went to the doctors as an emergency appointment because, in between heaving sobs that shook my body, I asked for help. I knew I deserved help for the sake of my loved ones. My sudden breakdown and suicidal feelings were obviously a concern and so my GP helped me look into why.

I had a Mirena coil fitted over 5 years ago. I was told, when it was fitted, that this would see me through the menopause and should last 10 years. In June 2023 we passed the five-year mark which is when the hormones stopped being released into my body. In the middle of July, I had a sudden hormone surge or dump, for want of a better word, and there was nothing in my system to counterbalance it. In other words, the full might of the menopause hit me square in the face, in the middle of a festival, and I felt so lost, so confused, so scared, so dreadful and so alien from myself that I wanted to die.

It terrifies me that this is happening up and down the country without women getting and receiving proper help. I was put straight on anti-depressants, which have helped enormously, and my GP took some blood tests to see what had gone on. To find out if you are in menopause your blood is tested for FSH (follicle-stimulating hormone). A level of 30 and over is a good indicator that you are menopausal. To quote my GP 'your level is well in excess of that.'

I had, unknowingly, been left with a defunct Mirena coil and a sudden huge influx or exodus, I'm not sure which, of hormones which sent my brain haywire and left me a panic-stricken shell of myself.

Too many of us are left to feel that we are alone in this fight. Times are changing but it is not happening quickly enough. My GP has now put me on HRT in the hope that my hormones balance out again.
But the list of side effects is terrifying.
Years ago, our life expectancy did not extend much beyond the childbearing years. But today we are living with our ovaries literally dying inside of us.
If men's bollocks shrivelled up and died between the ages of 48 and 56, do you really believe that they would be prescribed a drug with side effects such as blood clots, three different types of cancer, sickness, weight gain, migraines etc?

Do you believe they would be given misinformation and fobbed off, as I was, with near catastrophic results?

We, as women, deserve so much better than we are getting. Fight for yourself, fight for the right to live your life without wanting to end it. What we do today, as women, will pave the way for our daughters to have an easier, better time of it, so please, speak out if you are suffering and get the help you deserve.

Did I ball Sacks!

Tuesday, 12th September 2023

Last night I got in before my husband. Both daughters were away so we had the house to ourselves.

I ran upstairs to the bedroom, stripped off and….

Did I shit, shower, shave, floss, fake tan and dress alluringly in silk undies for my man, draping myself across the bed?

Did I ball sacks.

I sniffed my arm pits to see if they would go another couple of hours and put my pyjamas on.

It was 5 past five.

When David got in, he did exactly the same.

We cuddled up on the sofa, until the spaniel forcibly came between us, and watched TV.

These are the moments that make a marriage.

The sharing of space.

When you can scratch your bum, pick your nose, pluck your chin – not all at the same time, unless you are supremely lucky, think of the time you would save! – in your most comfortable pyjamas, in front of your partner and be completely yourself.

I am sure my husband would occasionally like to come home to find me draped alluringly across the bed in silk undies, but as a flap is likely to flop out of my French Knickers, or a bit of peed on gusset is always a possibility, the fantasy tends to be better than the reality.

I don't think I have a fantasy.

The thought of a good night's sleep without thunderous snoring and aggressive farting feels like a dream.

When I think of what turns me on, I think of David waving his lad in my face telling me the cure all will make my menopause better if only I would take it orally or have it rubbed on my chest. Hardly the stuff of fantasy, but it makes us laugh and that is sexy.

Maybe we are too comfortable with each other, but I enjoy this phase in our lives when we can just be very genuinely ourselves. After these last few years of menopause, when I have been up and down, raging, despairing, irrational and upset, when he has seen my shave my face and my arse, and when I am bloated and covered in sweat and, frankly, any hole can and does explode, there is little mystique left. Frequently in our house you will hear: 'David, get the mop, I've piddled again' or 'excuse me while I strip off and bundle my pants into the washing machine' or, my personal favourite: 'David, I've just shit myself climbing over the stair gate.'

I like that his eyes light up if I do make the effort to look nice. I know I have done well when he gets the same look on his face as when I make pork chop with stilton cheese sauce. Maybe tonight I will tuck my flaps into a little sexy something, leave the lube drawer open and aim for pork chop eyes.

Although he has just reminded me that he has a rotator cuff injury. I am not sure how this is relevant unless he thinking of rotating me on a rotisserie, like a spit roast?

Pyjamas it is then.

Happy ever after?

22nd September 2023

Last night, after nearly two weeks on the HRT, I looked at my husband's feet and felt a fanny twinge.

His Feet! For the love of Mary!

Even when we first got together, and I could not even look at him without my knickers falling off, I never once found his feet attractive.

The only feet I have ever liked were my babies tiny little, kissable feet.

Feet are gnarly, hairy, tough skinned, ugly hoofy parts of us that are not attractive in any way.

They are stuffed in socks and shoes and emerge smelling like something has gone off.

Yet, as husband stretched his bare feet towards me last night, expecting, no doubt, the usual 'get those cheesy trotters away from me' I found myself looking at them and thinking 'hmmm, bare, naked skin.'

My eyes travelled up his tartan pyjama clad legs (well, it was half past eight) and I licked my lips.

The fluttering feeling intensified, it felt vaguely familiar, like visiting a place you once went on holiday to or bumping into an old school friend.

The feet inched towards me, and I found myself wanting to reach out and touch them.

This goes against all my natural instincts, which would usually be to recoil in horror and leap off the sofa, but I felt powered on by a deep, primal instinct, more powerful than my revulsion.

I realised I felt horny.

My husband's feet were making me have sexual twinges.

Proof, if ever it was needed, that HRT is indeed a miracle drug.

I'll keep you posted.

One last thing…
Cut this out and keep it at work

How to help the menopausal woman in the workplace:
Get a fan
Get some tissues
Get a mop
Don't be young and thin
Praise the benefits of elasticated clothing
Install air conditioning
Let her deal with all the arsey customers – she will enjoy it
Pass the cold callers over to her, you will never hear from them again
Make the company motto: Sweaty women are sexy women
Use her to negotiate pay rises – management will be scared
Play brass band music in the background so she can fart in comfort and pass it off as a tuba
Smile encouragingly when she forgets what she is saying in the middle of saying it
Say 'oh but a flushed red face really suits you!'
Don't allow anyone into the office with a cold – sneezes are not her friend.
Encourage her to keep a voodoo doll to offset rage
Respect the fact that she knows her stuff, she has just temporarily forgotten it
Be kind to her, she is going through a really shitty time.